Drumming Asian America

Drumming Asian America

Taiko, Performance, and Cultural Politics

Angela K. Ahlgren

OXFORD
UNIVERSITY PRESS

OXFORD

UNIVERSITY PRESS

Oxford University Press is a department of the University of Oxford. It furthers
the University's objective of excellence in research, scholarship, and education
by publishing worldwide. Oxford is a registered trade mark of Oxford University
Press in the UK and certain other countries.

Published in the United States of America by Oxford University Press
198 Madison Avenue, New York, NY 10016, United States of America.

© Oxford University Press 2018

Library of Congress Cataloging-in-Publication Data
Name: Ahlgren, Angela K., author.
Title: Drumming Asian America : taiko, performance, and cultural politics / Angela K. Ahlgren.
Description: New York, NY : Oxford University Press, [2018] |
Includes bibliographical references and index.
Identifiers: LCCN 2017044638 (print) | LCCN 2017048117 (ebook) | ISBN 9780199374038 (updf) |
ISBN 9780199374014 (cloth : alk. paper) | ISBN 9780199374021 (pbk. : alk. paper)
Subjects: LCSH: Taiko (Drum ensemble)—United States. | Music—Social aspects—United States. |
Asian American musicians.
Classification: LCC ML1038.T35 (ebook) | LCC ML1038.T35 A55 2018 (print) |
DDC 786.9089/95073—dc23
LC record available at https://lccn.loc.gov/2017044638

9 8 7 6 5 4 3 2 1

Paperback printed by Webcom, Inc., Canada

Hardback printed by Bridgeport National Bindery, Inc., United States of America

For my sister
Jill Marie Ahlgren
1977–2013

CONTENTS

PREFACE

When I first began taking taiko classes, before we even pulled out our practice drums, we learned to move our bodies. Before we hit the drum, we needed to know the *kata*, the basic physical form, of taiko. First, we did a warm-up. Jumping jacks, three sets of ten, counted out loud in Japanese (*ichi, ni, san, shi . . .*). We swung our arms in wide circles to loosen our shoulders, we stretched our calves, and we rolled our wrists. The tape-wrapped tires mounted on folding chairs that served as practice drums remained on the periphery of the room. We stood in rows and learned how to align our feet, hips, torsos, and arms, orienting ourselves toward an imaginary instrument. We learned how to swing our arms toward the drum, one body part at a time: first the hips, then the belly, the elbow, the wrist, and finally the *bachi* (the drumsticks) moving toward the drumhead. Right, then left, right, then left. One, two, one, two. *Ichi, ni, ichi, ni.* This was "air taiko." Still the drums remained on the sidelines. We needed to absorb the choreography before we could make music.

Taiko is a form of ensemble drumming that originated in Japan in the early 1950s. It was taken up by Japanese Americans in the late 1960s in California and has become increasingly popular in recent decades in the United States, Canada, Europe, South America, and now in other parts of Asia. The first time I witnessed a taiko concert was in December 1998. I was twenty-two. In those days, I worked as a stage manager for Theater Mu, an Asian American theater company in Minneapolis whose artistic director, Rick Shiomi, had recently started a taiko group that would eventually become a major part of the organization. I was asked to fill in for the regular stage manager for one night of the group's second annual taiko concert at the Southern Theatre, a beloved Minneapolis venue with dilapidated, crumbling-brick charm. By 1998 taiko had already developed a large following in the United States, especially on the West Coast among Japanese American communities, but to this white woman in Minnesota, it was still brand new. The appealing unison movement, the rolling thunder of drumbeats, and the anticipation-filled space between beats (what I would come to know as *ma*) held my attention like no other performance.

One of the pieces that captivated me was "Pounding Hooves," a song written by Rick Shiomi that built speed through unison movement while allowing individual performers to distinguish themselves in solos. It started with a slow and sultry swing beat, one drummer, then two, then three, unfolding from bent knees with a flourish of outstretched arms, softly beating their rhythms on the large barrel-shaped taiko while a fourth drummer kept the *ji*, or base beat, on the upstage *shime-daiko* (high-pitched rope tension drum). Low martial-arts stances matched the angle of the drums, forty-five degrees. The left knee bent toward the audience and the right leg stretched long. After each drummer played a section introducing the song's major rhythms, the three finally cohered in unison sound and movement: three arms, three bachi, and three flashes of blue *happi* coat sleeve zinged toward and away from us on alternating beats. *Don! Don! Don! Don!* Arms reached for the heavens, and shouts animated the space between beats. At the crest of a crescendo the bachi cracked out a sharp "*ka, ka!*" on the rims of the drums as the drummers swept their arms down and around, propelling a turn to the other side of the drums. The seven beats of silence that occurred while the drummers' arms whooshed and their feet box-stepped around the drums filled the theater with anticipation. I watched carefully from my perch in the light booth, trying to discern the beginning of the next section in anticipation of the light cue. On the last silent beat of the *ma*, the drummers leapt into the air as they unfurled their arms, expanded their chests, and shouted "*HA!*" Their bachi landed on the drumheads as the drummers' feet reached the floor, and the moment was pure satisfaction.

Watching the six or so Asian American women and men move with such grace and power, I had no idea if this was something white people did. Yet I was moved to find out. About three minutes into the song the solos began, and my eyes were drawn to Jen on the stage-left drum as she burst into her solo with fierce joy. No longer constrained by the song's choreography, she threw herself into every strike of the drum and every fling of her arm with intense abandon. A Korean American woman five feet, two inches tall, Jen was transformed before me, larger than life. She leapt to face the drum head-on and lifted her face to the audience, opening her mouth in a silent roar as she beat an X-pattern on the drumhead before spinning around and laying out the rhythm that signaled the end of her solo. Two more solos followed, electric and graceful. I understand now that the performers had been playing for only a few years, but that night their artistry transformed me.

Most taiko players I know have a version of this love-at-first-sight story: they saw taiko and wanted to play. This is mine, and it is shot through with both the pleasure of watching women perform and wanting to perform alongside them. Virtuosity, as performance ethnographer Judith Hamera writes, organizes the performer and the spectator into a social relationship propelled by "the power of the vicarious."[1] Describing the performer Oguri's dances, Hamera writes, "The effects are more than visually arresting; they invite visceral, corporeal empathy."[2] Watching Mu Daiko from the tech booth, I responded kinesthetically to the performance. I wanted to be able to do what the drummers were doing. Their power and fluidity seemed unattainable, and I had no sense that I could achieve such feats of artistry and athleticism. And yet I wanted to. It looked effortless but also impossibly difficult—athletic, musical, powerful, beautiful, larger than life. Something about the joyful ferocity with which the drummers propelled themselves into and around those drums was appealing on a gut level.

With the emphasis on gesture and large-scale choreographed movement that is part of this musical practice, taiko lends itself to—indeed, requires—thinking about music and dance together. Taiko thus makes manifest the troubling of boundaries and the slipping out from under definitions that is also central to inquiries of racial, gender, and sexual identity, questions I explore in this book. Some taiko players see themselves as musicians, others as movers, and still others as simply and only taiko players. Taiko is music and dance, music-as-dance, or as longtime taiko player Jeanne Mercer puts it, "music in motion."[3] Many kinds of music making might be read as dance because, in the words of ethnomusicologist Matthew Rahaim, "[W]hen people make music, they move: a finger slides along the neck of a violin, a palm whacks a drumhead, a laryngeal cartilage tilts back and forth as air is pushed through the vocal folds."[4] In other words, there can be no music making without movement somewhere in the body. In taiko, as in other musical genres, the body moves and sounds simultaneously; without movement, sound would be impossible. But taiko is both things together, music-as-dance, in a way that not all musical practices are. Drums are configured in different patterns for each piece, and the drum placement facilitates a variety of movements and choreographies. While some movements are simply a matter of producing sound (the arm must move up or back in order to create enough force to produce the resounding *don* on the drumhead), others are designed to create stunning visual effects or to emphasize the musculature of the player's body. Each piece, in other words, is choreographed in terms of both creating stage pictures through the arrangement and locomotion of performers and through the performers' moving their own bodies while they play. Rahaim calls the music-making body in motion a "musicking body."[5] Taiko bodies are both musicking and dancing, sounding and moving bodies, as well as sensual and sensing bodies.

It is this combination of music and motion that produces such undeniable kinesthetic effects on taiko audiences and performers alike. It was, in part, its impossible-to-ignore sonic and visual qualities that made taiko so appealing to Asian Americans in the late 1960s and 1970s, and later bolstered efforts to challenge prevailing stereotypes of Asians as quiet and passive.[6] Recent data collection efforts by the Taiko Community Alliance show that women comprise roughly 64 percent of North American taiko players who responded to their survey, and the genre's feminist appeal is well documented.[7] Still, often its embodiment of masculine power has been put to heteronormative and nationalistic use, and though women make up the majority of players, in many cases it is men who emerge as the stars of taiko (see Chapters 4 and 5).[8] This book attends to the ways choreographed movements relate to social movements and the ways musicking bodies also become bodies politic. I explore how taiko enables feminist, queer, and cross-racial intimacies, thus locating political potential not only in explicitly activist contexts but also in the erotic and the everyday.

When I first encountered Mu Daiko from the tech booth in 1998 the ensemble was comprised of beginners, but to me their performance represented something completely beyond the scope of my abilities—and beyond the bounds of whiteness. Describing her first encounters with taiko from her perspective as an Asian American woman Deborah Wong writes, "I had been moved many times by Asian American music-making, but watching taiko was one long extended moment of wanting to *do* that, wanting to *be* that—a deep urgent desire that I can now only describe as a truly performative effect. Watching taiko made me want to do it and all that that means."[9] What Wong hints at but does not quite say is that her experience of watching taiko was erotic, a kind of kinesthetic experience that urged her to move and to act on the desires the drumming instilled. Her double entendre, "made me want to do it and all that that means," indicates an urge both to play taiko and to satisfy erotic desires. As it was for Wong, my first experience with taiko was a deeply visceral and sensual experience that was wrapped up in wanting to do what the performers were doing, to be with them, particularly the women, and to be what they simply *were*: strong, graceful, and unfettered.

Taiko did not answer a call to know my racial identity in the same way it has for Wong and other Asian American taiko players. In that first encounter, thinking about the small group of Asian American performers before me, I wondered if it would be audacious for a white person to think about joining the group. Did white people play taiko? At that time, my question was not one of cultural appropriation or white privilege but about observing the boundaries of a company with a specific mission to create work by and for Asian Americans. Mu Daiko was part of a theater company dedicated to creating roles for Asian American actors and producing plays by Asian American playwrights. It would have seemed perfectly reasonable that the group would also prioritize the development of Asian American taiko players. But it offered classes that were open to the public. Within a month of that first concert, I took my first taiko class. A year later I—along with several other new players—was performing on the stage of the Southern Theater with Mu Daiko. Between 1999 and 2009 I took classes and workshops, became an intern and then a performing member of Mu Daiko, taught classes, composed a taiko performance, and generally immersed myself in taiko as my primary passion.

Over time, my understanding of my own racial identity would be profoundly shaped by taiko and the relationships built in practicing it, but these insights came later. Taiko is a practice I share with a great number of Asian Americans, and often performances situate me alongside them on stage. It is from my position as a white, queer bisexual woman that I witness the everyday racism, Orientalism, and rapt curiosity that audiences bring to Asian American performance. It is also where I have experienced the instances of transformation, inspiration, and cross-racial intimacies that taiko can enable. Performance requires participants to put their bodies on the line, to be recognized or misrecognized, to be subject to critique, evaluation, or adoration. This book is an act of witnessing, an "interactive" response to the ways race, gender, and sexuality are bound up in the performances that take place on stage and off.[10]

Taiko brings people together not only on stage but also in activities like sweating together in rehearsal, packing up equipment in an unscripted choreography, and enjoying beer and sushi while rehashing the mistakes and triumphs of a performance. Perhaps all forms of performance-making enable these kinds of communion, but this book foregrounds the space taiko has made for such intimacies. What Hamera says of dancers is true for taiko players, too: performers "reach across multiple dimensions of difference to incarnate new shared aesthetic and social possibilities."[11] Taiko players in North America often describe themselves as part of a community, even a family. And yet the rehearsal space, the theater, and the myriad other spaces in which taiko players gather are never free from hierarchies, disputes, and inequities. This book moves through these spaces and rehearses the possibilities in taiko performance.

ACKNOWLEDGMENTS

Much like taiko, scholarship comes to life as part of a community. Far from a solitary process, writing this book happened in the company of others: not only those whose performances and rehearsals I attended but also peers and friends who shaped and challenged my thinking, mentors who supported my scholarship, and colleagues across disciplines and institutions who read and responded to drafts and ideas.

My research was made possible by support from a number of institutions and organizations. A Continuing Fellowship from the University of Texas at Austin allowed me to finish my work in a timely manner, faculty research funds from Ohio University supported travel to conduct interviews, and awards from the American Society for Theatre Research (ASTR) and the Congress on Research in Dance (CORD) allowed me to develop the work by attending national conferences. Of particular importance was the inaugural Mellon Dance Studies in/and the Humanities institute at Northwestern University in 2012. The colleagues and mentors I met there have made all the difference in ushering this book forward and in shaping my scholarship and commitment to dance, broadly construed, as a key mode of scholarly inquiry. Norm Hirschy at Oxford University Press guided me through my first book with patience and openness, and the anonymous manuscript reviewers provided crucial insights that shaped the final work for the better.

The faculty of Performance as Public Practice at the University of Texas at Austin, in particular, Jill Dolan, Charlotte Canning, and Deborah Paredez, nurtured the dissertation version of this project. Beyond that, the feminist, queer, and antiracist work of the faculty and students of PPP (past and present) continues to reverberate in my life in important ways. But this project actually started earlier, as two different papers in Asian American Studies graduate seminars at the University of Minnesota. Josephine Lee's Asian American Cultural Critique class and Erika Lee's Asian American History class inspired the questions and initial writings that became part of a master's degree portfolio and, later, the dissertation. The confluence of my Asian American Studies coursework at Minnesota and my experiences with Theater Mu and Mu Daiko formed an important basis for what came later.

What appears in these pages was shaped by the insights and support of colleagues in formal and informal writing groups. My work is sharper and smarter thanks to the critical generosity of Rosemary Candelario, Hannah Kosstrin, Eleanor Owicki, Leonardo Cardoso, Kim Kattari, Kareem Khubchandani, Rumya Putcha, Vanita Reddy, Clare Croft, Jessica del Vecchio, Shelley Manis, Michelle Dvoskin, Jacob Juntunen, and Jonathan Chambers, members of the PPP dissertation writing group at the University of Texas at Austin, and the Performance and Culture Research Group at the Glasscock Center of Texas A&M University. A special thank you goes to Hannah Kosstrin for reading the manuscript at a critical stage and providing me with thoughtful feedback. For inviting me to present parts of this book in formal presentations and classroom discussions, I thank Harmony Bench and the Ohio State University Humanities Institute, Lei Ouyang Bryant and Skidmore College, Bill Condee and the School of Interdisciplinary Arts at Ohio University, Julie Iezzi and the University of Hawaii at Manoa, Kathy Meizel and the College of Musical Arts at Bowling Green State University, Petra Kuppers and the English Department at the University of Michigan, and Angela Kane and the Dance Colloquium at the University of Michigan.

For their mentorship and collegial support while I balanced finishing the manuscript with faculty responsibilities, I am grateful to Bill Condee at Ohio University; Kirsten Pullen and Donnalee Dox at Texas A&M University; and Jonathan Chambers, Cynthia Baron, and Lesa Lockford at Bowling Green State University. The keen research assistance and transcription skills of Rebecca Hammonds kept this book on track in its later stages.

I am fortunate to be developing this work among people whose scholarship and embodied practice of taiko yield wide-ranging and fascinating insights. Lei Ouyang Bryant, Benjamin Pachter, Kate Walker, Deborah Wong, and Paul Yoon have proved to be lively interlocutors. In particular, Deborah Wong and Lei Ouyang Bryant have helped me think about taiko as Asian Americanist and feminist praxis. Though we have only communicated electronically, Paul Yoon has influenced my work through his scholarship and by founding a taiko group at Bowling Green State University that I now have the privilege of teaching and advising. Since early in my graduate work, Deborah Wong has been an enthusiastic, supportive, and gracious mentor and colleague. This book is all the better for her generous reading of the manuscript and for the superb taiko scholarship she has been producing for many years.

Working with Theater Mu and Mu Daiko attuned me to new modes of thinking about identity, about communities, and about what performance can do in the world. Whether their names appear here or not, each member, leader, and student of Mu Daiko, and the hours spent sweating in the rehearsal space, performing together, and driving to gigs across Minnesota, inspired this book. I still miss teaching the Saturday morning class and hanging out in the dressing rooms at the Southern Theater. For reading and responding to chapter drafts I thank Jennifer Weir, Heewon Lee, Su-Yoon Ko, and Rachel Gorton. During my years with the group, Rick Shiomi, Iris Shiraishi, and Jennifer Weir formed a dynamic trio of leadership, inspiration, and support, and I cannot quantify the ways in which each of them has influenced this book.

Members of San Jose Taiko, Sacramento Taiko Dan, Jodaiko, Odaiko Sonora, the Great Lakes Taiko Center, Soten Taiko, and Kogen Taiko gave their time and insights in interviews, all of which made this book possible. For giving their time and insights to the interview process and for allowing me to incorporate them into this book, thank you to Amanda, Gregg Amundson, Yurika Chiba, Jeff Ellsworth, Kenny Endo, Rachel Gorton, Naomi Guilbert, P. J. Hirabayashi, Roy Hirabayashi, Franco Imperial, Eileen Kage, Su-Yoon Ko, Faye Komagata, Shuji Komagata, Leslie Komori, Susie Kuniyoshi, Heewon Lee, Sascha Molina, Alan Okada, Kristy Oshiro, Rick Shiomi, Iris Shiraishi, Tanis Sotelo, Nicole Stansbury, Meg Suzuki, Tiffany Tamaribuchi, Wisa Uemura, Adam Weiner, Jennifer Weir, David Wells, Toyomi Yoshida, Shereen Youngblood, and Al Zdrazil. Not every person's words made it to the final manuscript, but everyone's insights shaped my thinking.

I also thank Austin Taiko and UT Gindaiko at the University of Texas at Austin for allowing me, a stranger, to join them on occasion and to borrow their equipment. Thank you to photographers Charissa Uemura, Katharine Saunders, Jeanie Ow, Higashi Design, Ray Yuen, and Drew Gorton, for sharing their artistry and allowing me to make it part of the book. I am also grateful to the Taiko Community Alliance and the TCA Census Committee (now the Tech Committee) for allowing me to join them, for helping me get the data I needed, and for undertaking the labor of conducting a census. Thank you to Wisa Uemura of San Jose Taiko and Shannon Freeby of Mu Performing Arts for helping me track down photos and other organizational information. Finally, thank you to the organizers and participants at the 2017 Women and Taiko gathering for reinvigorating my enthusiasm for practicing this art form.

My family faced much sorrow during the years when I was writing this book. Through it, my parents, Bruce and Marla Ahlgren, and my brother Jonathan encouraged and supported me, seeing me through job searches and multiple cross-country moves, all the while urging me to keep writing. Before she died in 2013, my sister Jill shared with me her excitement that I was writing a book and always offered me humor, love, and her infectious positive thinking. My grandmother, Rachel Maki, shared her home with me for two summers, and I reaped the considerable benefits of her company, her love, and her home cooking. Just for existing in the world as their beautiful selves I thank my niece and nephew, Aili Huhta and Kai Huhta. The eternally patient Sam has supported and encouraged me through the final, but what nevertheless feel like endless, stages of writing a book. And Meg Hanna Tominaga knows exactly when to offer me serious moral support or ridiculous made-up songs. For this and many other reasons, her friendship is beyond compare. The love of my family and friends, those listed here and many others, make my work and my life (so deeply intertwined) possible and pleasurable.

I am grateful to Women and Performance, the University of Wisconsin Press, and Oxford University Press for granting permission to include previously published material in this book.

CHAPTER 1

Introduction

Drumming Asian America, Performing Cultural Politics

Taiko players make noise, move their bodies, shout and sweat. Often in unison, sometimes alone, they make themselves seen and heard on concert stages and at community festivals, corporate events, marches, and protests. Taiko audiences feel the drumbeats in their bodies as they watch and listen to the performers, most often Asian Americans, making music before them. This book is about the myriad ways in which North American taiko players perform Asian America and engage cultural politics from the late 1960s to the 2010s. It deals not only with the ways Asian Americans in various taiko groups perform identity within and alongside communities and social movements, but also with how taiko players from other or overlapping identity positions—white, black, feminist, and queer—participate in the racial formation of Asian America through taiko performance. *Drumming Asian America* asks what cultural, political, and aesthetic forces motivate performance choices, undergird group dynamics, and shape encounters between performers and their audiences. It asks how the mundane and the everyday perform politics alongside the spectacular and the staged. Examining the cultural politics entwined in the practice and performance of North American taiko enables new understandings of race, gender, and sexuality in and around Asian America.

Growing from just two groups in the late 1960s to around 200 groups by 2000 and more than 450 in 2016, North American taiko has exploded in popularity in a few short decades. A recent census of taiko players conducted by the Taiko Community Alliance, an organization whose mission it is to "empower the people and advance the art of taiko," counted 464 groups in the U.S. and Canada alone, more than double the estimated number when I began playing taiko in 1999.[1] This art form, therefore, warrants focused critical attention. In Japan, taiko is even more commonplace, with estimates of amateur and regional groups in the thousands and a number of highly visible professional touring ensembles such as Kodo, Ondekoza, Shidara, and Hono-O-Daiko. Shawn Bender's book *Taiko Boom* accounts for the cultural significance and popularity of ensemble drumming in postwar Japan, joining other English-language publications about Japanese taiko. And while this book constitutes the first scholarly monograph to focus on taiko in North America, it builds on essays, book chapters, and dissertations published by Deborah Wong, Paul Yoon, Masumi Izumi, Benjamin Pachter, and others who have illuminated the cultural, political, and aesthetic dimensions of the art form as it has developed in the late twentieth and twenty-first centuries.

This study does not attempt to map the entire taiko community, nor can it speak for every taiko player's experience. Rather, this book uses ethnographic and historical methods, alongside detailed performance analysis, to demonstrate the ways taiko as a physical practice rehearses social values and, in the words of Judith Hamera, "incarnate[s] new shared aesthetic and social possibilities."[2] The book takes taiko seriously as performance-making and community-building, with all of the complexities and debates they entail. My focus on Minnesota taiko in Chapter 3 and Midwestern performers in Chapter 4 highlights the Midwest as a key site for Asian American cultural production, a move that addresses the coastal bias of Asian American Studies and performance-related fields (figure 1.1). Similarly, by leveraging my position as a white woman taiko player, I examine how whiteness and blackness are constelled in Asian American performance and as racial categories in the United States. I also explore the ways taiko can be

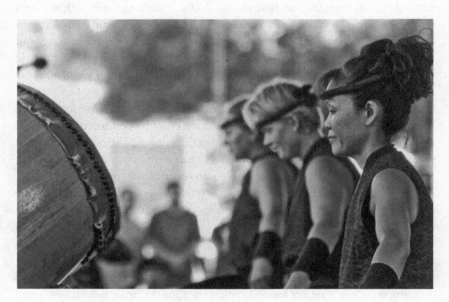

Figure 1.1. Mu Daiko members wait to perform at the Powell Street Festival, Vancouver, British Columbia, 2006. Photo by Jeanie Ow. Used with permission.

queered, not only by the presence of queer-identified performers on stage but also by acknowledging and enjoying the erotic aspects of taiko. Thus, when I contend that North American taiko players perform Asian America, I attempt not to circumscribe what Asian America is but rather to push against the edges of the category and to demonstrate the myriad ways taiko players embody it in and through performance.

Rather than champion taiko as simply liberatory or "just fun" (a sentiment espoused by many practitioners), I focus on the complex intersections among identities, communities, and ideologies that taiko puts into practice. Throughout the 1960s and 1970s, taiko presented a clear challenge to pervasive images of Asians as weak, silent, and passive. How have the politics and semiotics of taiko shifted in the 1990s and the early twenty-first century as more and more non-Asian Americans practice and perform in taiko groups? How have women and sexual minorities harnessed the political potential of taiko? Who belongs in the taiko community and on stage? What does it mean to "perform Asian America" in an allegedly post-racial nation whose urgent racial conflicts are framed as black-white issues? *Drumming Asian America* argues that North American taiko players complicate and challenge what it means to do so by commemorating Asian American histories, challenging gender and racial formations, inviting queer spectatorship, and engaging in a range of encounters with presenters, audiences, and each other.

At the same time as I propose that taiko is more than just fun, this book also recognizes the deep pleasures of taiko practice and performance and indeed the pleasures of the art form as a site for critical inquiry. Through detailed descriptions of performances, including the contexts surrounding them—rehearsal, performance sites, and encounters with audiences—I attempt to approximate for readers an experience of practicing, performing, watching, and listening to taiko. Although text is my medium in this book, I describe and analyze taiko not as a series of static texts but, to borrow from Ramón Rivera-Servera, as events and as "lived experience . . . inclusive of the audiences" whose presence contributes to the process of performance.[3] Even for fully staged concerts, backstage areas and dressing rooms, performers' nerves, sweat, and excitement all comprise the event, as do performers' strategic choices and audiences' reactions during and after performances. Rehearsals, drum-making, post-show meals, and the pressures of daily life also inform what taiko is and what it means. All of these (and more) become potential sites of pleasure, debate, compromise, and critical reflection. When I invoke the term "cultural politics," my primary concerns center on the triad of race, gender, and sexuality not as essential qualities but as processes informed by historical and cultural factors. Aesthetic codes and choices are thus only part of what this book is about, as I employ taiko as not only an object of study but also a lens though which to understand the constellation of social movements, racial formations, and embodied choreographies that approximate Asian American performance and cultural politics.

Taiko means "drum" or "fat drum" in Japanese. In this book, "taiko" refers to the ensemble drumming that developed in Japan in the 1950s and spread to the Americas, Europe, other parts of Asia, and Australia in subsequent decades. Some instrumentation used in taiko performance comes from Shinto and Buddhist rituals[4] or from Japanese performance traditions such as *gagaku* (court music) and Noh and Kabuki *bayashi* (musical accompaniment for Noh and Kabuki theater), but modern taiko distinguishes itself from these other practices by making the drumming the focus of performance, rather than an accompaniment to dance, theater, ritual, or festival activities. Sometimes scholars and practitioners use the term *kumi-daiko*, "group drumming," to differentiate the contemporary form from other Japanese percussion practices. *Wadaiko* is a term used in Japan to make a similar distinction. Other scholars use "kumi-daiko" or "wadaiko" when they are writing about drumming in a Japanese context and therefore require a different level of specificity. Because this book focuses on North America, where confusion over various kinds of Japanese drumming is rarely an issue, the term "taiko" suffices. But more than that, I write this book as a taiko player, and "taiko" is the word most North American taiko players use to refer to this art form.

Taiko is a twentieth-century phenomenon, but it is often painted as an ancient form both by players and by people marketing taiko performances. As a performer in Mu Daiko, I grew accustomed to telling audiences that in ancient Japan, taiko were used to communicate battle strategies in times of war, that the sound of taiko demarcated the boundaries of towns (if you could no longer hear the drum, you were beyond the town's limits), and that taiko were used to celebrate harvests or drive away evil spirits. Heidi Varian writes in her book *The Way of Taiko*, "Most villages had at least one drum, and its various rhythms were used for all aspects of everyday life. The drum was used to gather townspeople or warn of danger. It was beaten to signal war and send samurai into battle. Drummed messages could be sent across great distances in the village. Farmers would take the drums to the fields and drive pests from the crops or awaken the spirit of rain."[5] Varian's written account of taiko's past mirrors the many spoken accounts that draw on notions of an ancient agrarian Japan.[6] As ethnomusicologist Paul Yoon astutely observes, contemporary Japanese and American taiko groups "often emphasize (or more specifically, construct and imagine) the taiko's role in premodern Japanese life by highlighting the 'ancient' or 'authentic' roots of the music or musical endeavor."[7] Yoon's parenthetical statement that these accounts are constructed reveals his skepticism about their veracity. These accounts, which to my knowledge are largely unsupported, construct an idyllic and rural Japanese past that, when related in an American context, risk casting Japanese culture as permanently ancient and primitive.

Taiko is neither a wholly ancient nor a purely Japanese practice. Rather, it is both modern and hybrid in origin.[8] The form began to emerge against the backdrop of a rapidly industrializing postwar Japan. Two separate groups, both considered to have marked the beginning of this new tradition, began using traditional drums in new ways. Sukeroku Taiko (and later Oedo Sukeroku Taiko), based in Tokyo, was formed by several drummers known for their solo drumming at festivals.[9] They combined movement and festival drumming in a way that made the taiko itself the focus of performance. At about the same time, Daihachi Oguchi, a jazz drummer, arranged several differently pitched and sized Japanese drums to create complex rhythms. He combined traditional Japanese instrumentation with an American jazz drum configuration to create this new style of drumming. The group he formed is called O-Suwa Daiko.[10] These two groups, which had a significant impact on North American taiko, combined new traditions with old instruments and played Japanese music that was influenced by American musical idioms. As Jennifer Matsue contends, "[S]ince its inception taiko has been rooted in a multiplicity of cosmopolitan musical practices and innovative technique."[11] Claims about taiko's antiquity or its Japanese purity, thus, should be met with skepticism.

Taiko is also a transnational and global practice that encompasses myriad connections between drummers in Japan, the United States and Canada, the United Kingdom, Europe, Australia, and other parts of Asia. Facilitating many of these connections and exchanges over the course of nearly twenty years has been the North American Taiko Conference. Held every two years between 1997 and 2011 and again in 2015 and 2017, NATC brings together taiko practitioners from the United States and Canada, guest teachers from Japan, and attendees (albeit in smaller numbers) from Europe and other areas of the world.[12] The primary sponsor for the 2015 conference was the newly formed Taiko Community Alliance, a non-profit organization founded and run by taiko players after the long-time sponsor, the Japanese American Community and Cultural Center of Los Angeles, decided to focus on other efforts. Other regional and collegiate taiko conferences and gatherings are sometimes held in the interim years between national conferences, and 2014 marked the first World Taiko Gathering, held in Los Angeles.

Though it is a relatively recent phenomenon, taiko encompasses a wide variety of practices, instruments, musical influences, philosophies, and sets of etiquette and therefore requires a multidimensional critical approach. Capturing what taiko is in practice can be tricky because any given performance may entail much more than what can be conveyed in a basic definition. Even veteran players resist defining the form in terms of traditional genres.[13] This book focuses on contemporary taiko, which I venture to define as a physically demanding form of ensemble drumming that uses large barrel drums, as well as other rope-tensioned drums and percussion accessories, in performances that employ choreographed movement, often loosely based on martial arts stances and moves. Yet the groups I write about exceed this definition, since they draw on multiple dance forms and musical styles. And some of the pieces I focus on, such as P. J. Hirabayashi's taiko folk dance "Ei Ja Nai Ka?," combine dance with drumming, flute, and vocals.

If taiko resists categorization as a genre, neither can taiko be adequately addressed within a single discipline. With its emphasis on visual arrangement and choreography, taiko is particularly suited to choreographic analysis, yet its sonic dimensions cannot be ignored. It is performance that asks us to think about how musicians move, how movers sound, and how these movements and sounds together stage and articulate a variety of identitarian, communitarian, and political stances. In this book I attend to the corporeal, the choreographic, and the sensual aspects of taiko and ask how these movements activate a variety of cultural, political, and personal ends. I therefore draw on scholarship from disciplines including dance studies, ethnomusicology, performance studies, and theater history to think through how taiko makes meaning.

Taiko is thus much more complex than its simplest definition as Japanese drumming might indicate. It is a global form that is often tied to local communities; it is a marker of postwar Japanese nationality and late twentieth-century Asian American identity; it is an art form with evolving conventions and aesthetic codes; it is a leisure activity, a form of exercise, and for some, a spiritual practice; it is music, dance, and theater; and it is a social practice that, in North America, has a great deal of overlap with Asian American history, activism, community, and performance.

BECOMING ASIAN AMERICAN, PERFORMING POLITICS

The cover of William Wei's book *The Asian American Movement* features an image of a single taiko player and her drum in front of a banner that reads, "Coalition to Commemorate Vincent Chin." One can imagine the onlookers listening to the somber—or perhaps angry—rhythms of this taiko player as they gather to remember the Chinese American man whose beating death at the hands of two white auto workers in Detroit in 1981 and their scant punishments sparked outrage among Asian American activists. Although Wei's book never mentions taiko as a politically engaged art form, images such as this one demonstrate that taiko players have indeed lent their talents to protests, commemorations, and other politically motivated gatherings. Since its earliest years in the United States, taiko has been performed in contexts that celebrate Japanese American community, stake out emergent Asian American identities, and protest racist policies and human rights violations. Today it is possible to see taiko not only at Japanese and Asian American memorials such as days of remembrance commemorating Japanese internment but also in LGBTQ pride parades and other such cultural and political celebrations not solely tied to Asian or Asian American communities. In the summer of 2016, for example, both Soh Daiko of New York and Mu Daiko of Minneapolis issued LGBT pride edition t-shirts, with their group logos in rainbow-colored text. In a recent post on the Taiko Community Facebook group, one player expressed a desire to use taiko to contribute to such current social justice efforts as Black Lives Matter; other groups performed at the many women's marches across the United States following the 2017 presidential inauguration.

In the late 1960s, North American taiko players, along with a host of other activists and organizations, began to articulate what "Asian American" meant. The first two U.S. taiko groups, San Francisco Taiko Dojo and Kinnara Taiko of Los Angeles, formed in 1968 and 1969 respectively, amid a broader context of social change for Japanese American communities influenced by the civil rights and black power movements and by antiwar activism and a newly coalescing Asian American identity. Los Angeles and San Francisco were major centers of activity not only for the Asian American movement but also for Japanese American community organizing.

Before this period the political organizing of Asians in the United States was for the most part based on ethnic, rather than racial, commonalities. According to Wei, in the wake of the civil rights era, many Asian Americans came together with the realization that they were "*in* American culture, but not of it." Protests during the Vietnam War spurred the formation of pan-Asian coalitions. Many Americans of Asian descent had been involved in feminist, New Left, and civil rights activism, but antiwar activism "brought them together psychologically and politically."[14] As Glenn Omatsu writes, the student strikes at San Francisco State College and the University of California at Berkeley, organized under the auspices of the Third World Liberation Front, not only resulted in the implementation of ethnic studies courses in those universities but also "critically transformed the consciousness of its participants," whose actions echoed those of earlier activist movements. These student activists "reclaimed a heritage of struggle" set forth by "earlier generations of Pilipino farm workers, Chinese immigrant garment and restaurant workers, and Japanese American concentration camp resisters."[15] The widespread establishment of social services organizations among Asian American communities followed Mao's "power to the people" philosophy and the Black Panther Party's "serve the people" approach.[16] In 1969 a conference at the University of California at Berkeley called "Asian American Experience in America—Yellow Identity" attempted to create a sense of pan-Asian solidarity among mainly Chinese and Japanese American student groups.[17] Activists in the movement were inspired by both civil rights organizing and the black power movement. Many Japanese Americans in Los Angeles in the postwar years were culturally and politically informed by their experiences growing up in largely black neighborhoods.[18] Movement activists were also inspired by peoples' uprisings in Asia, Africa, and Latin America and opposed U.S. imperialism.[19]

In addition to student strikes and the formation of service organizations, the Asian American movement included cultural dimensions, with some members working under the Maoist philosophy that artists were also cultural workers creating art "for the people."[20] Musicians, writers, and performers began to create artworks as individuals and as organizations. The folk trio A Grain of Sand performed at activist events and college campuses around the nation, and the title of their 1973 album, *A Grain of Sand: Music for the Struggle by Asians in America*, positions them squarely within the movement.[21] Jazz musician Fred Ho created music that was explicitly for and about Asian American experiences and causes. In 1970 the short-lived Asian American publication *Aion* published its two issues, which included writing and artwork that bespoke the need for activism.[22] Similarly, the magazine *Gidra*, which ran from 1969 to 1974, covered issues related to Asian American activism, identity, and community.[23] Not only did taiko groups form at around the same time, but several taiko players in pioneer groups moved in the activist, musical, and literary circles mentioned here.

In addition to these musicians' and writers' works, the 1960s and 1970s saw the founding of several theater companies and organizations dedicated to providing work for Asian American actors. These theater companies were not officially part of the Asian American movement, but they were part of a cultural shift toward adopting the term "Asian American" as an alternative to "Oriental." Through theater, actors once considered Oriental began to mine their own experiences to produce works by and about themselves as Asian Americans. In 1965 several actors of Asian descent in Hollywood (including Mako, Beulah Quo, Soon Tek-Oh, and Pat Li) founded East-West Players, a group initially dedicated to showcasing their talent to Hollywood agents. Eventually, the company's efforts turned increasingly toward developing acting talent as well as nurturing plays written by and about Asian Americans.[24] In 1968 actors organized under the name Oriental Actors of America to protest the casting of white actors in Asian roles.[25] These musical, literary, and theatrical efforts contested their racialization as Orientals and moved toward a new paradigm, Asian American.

Alongside these artists and activists, taiko groups forming in the late 1960s and early 1970s similarly explored what it meant to be Asian American. But this shift toward a pan-Asian coalition did not erase and has not erased Japanese or Japanese American identity from taiko, nor has it limited participation in taiko to those who identify as Asian American. It is important to acknowledge that, as Deborah Wong writes, "the slippage between taiko as a specifically Japanese performance tradition, to its emergence as a Japanese American tradition, to its reformulation as a pan-Asian American tradition, to its placement as a tradition open to any participants from any background, is central to the place of taiko in America."[26] In the earliest years, taiko players were exploring taiko as Japanese, as Japanese American, and as Asian American. I return to the specific ways the first three North American taiko groups (known among taiko players as the pioneer groups) negotiated these issues below.

If the form has become "open to participants from any background," why approach taiko through an Asian Americanist lens? The first answer is that Asian Americans, including those who identify as mixed-race, comprise approximately 60 percent of North American taiko players.[27] Not all of them necessarily practice for reasons related to identity, but in terms of percentage, taiko is clearly Asian American. But this perspective is not about quantifying an Asian American presence in taiko. More urgently, focusing on racial (as well as gendered and sexual) dimensions of taiko nuances racial politics in the United States, which continues to be framed in mainstream media as a black-white issue, despite the centrality of Asians to definitions of race early in the country's history.

Owing in part to the ways Asian Americans have been alternately racialized as ethnic outsiders *and* as model minorities, they often are not seen as part of the United States' problem of racism.[28] This attitude has been borne out in my classroom when I have taught Asian American theater courses. Students, mostly white, routinely learn for the first time that there is such a thing as anti-Asian racism. The history of taiko in the United States is intimately bound up with histories of anti-Asian racism, exclusion, incarceration, and broader civil rights struggles of the late twentieth century. Taiko illuminates histories of Asian American activism and contemporary racist attitudes at the same time as it highlights the work of Asian American artists and centers the bodies and voices of Asian American performers. Furthermore, apprehending the body in performance bridges the political and the performative, since both performance and activism require participants to show up and put their bodies on the line to achieve their ends.

While performers of many races are increasingly drawn to taiko, this book centers Asian American artists in all but one chapter. Dance scholars Yutian Wong and Priya Srinivasan have demonstrated the ways American dance history depends on narratives of white innovation to the exclusion of the Asian American artists who contributed to the work of such early choreographer-performers as Loie Fuller, Ruth St. Denis, and Martha Graham.[29] Taiko is an immensely popular form the majority of whose practitioners in North America are Asian American. Although white and other non-Asian performers participate at all levels, they have by no means eclipsed the work of Asian American performers, teachers, and leaders. Thus, this project provides an opportunity to consider issues of appropriation and racial politics not in recovery or revisionist mode, excavating the work of early innovators from underneath the fame of white performers, but on the ground as the form develops.

PIONEERING TAIKO: A BRIEF HISTORY OF EASTWARD EXPANSION

From its earliest years in the United States, taiko emerged as an art form practiced primarily by Japanese Americans and Japanese nationals. People who were not of Japanese descent also participated, but the three first groups, San Francisco Taiko Dojo, Kinnara Taiko, and San Jose Taiko, formed within specific local Japanese American contexts. To different degrees, each group was influenced by the emerging Asian American movement, but all were dependent on local Japanese American institutions. From there, groups began to form elsewhere in California, the West Coast of Canada, and eventually in the Midwest and the East Coast.

The San Francisco Taiko Dojo, led by Seiichi Tanaka, formed in San Francisco in 1968. Although many Japanese American taiko players, in particular, those who had been raised in Los Angeles and the Bay Area, may have been shaped by a lifetime of urban segregation and domestic racism, Tanaka arrived in California as an immigrant from Japan in 1967. Japan experienced student protests and radical demonstrations in the 1960s, but nothing in Tanaka's interviews or public statements connects him to those radical movements. Tanaka was in his early twenties when he came to the United States; he was, as a first-generation immigrant (*issei*), about the same age as most *sansei*, or third-generation Japanese Americans. He is considered *shin-issei*, a Japanese national who emigrated once the U.S. government eased restrictions on Japanese immigration after World War II. Tanaka's articulations of his goals for performing and teaching taiko resonate more with assimilationist than with radical politics. For example, according to his group's Web site, Tanaka "dreamed that the word 'taiko,' like 'karate' and 'sushi,' would one day become an integral part of the American vocabulary."[30] Nonetheless, members of his group were engaged in political activity, and Tanaka occasionally lent his talents to political situations he cared about.[31]

The story of Seiichi Tanaka's founding of the San Francisco Taiko Dojo is one that many taiko players know well: the origin story emphasizes Tanaka's status as an immigrant and his direct access to Japanese taiko experts.[32] Alongside Tanaka's legendary personality and his vision of making taiko a household word, a number of community institutions and dedicated practitioners helped build what is now a major performing arts company and school. These early connections tie the group to local Japanese American institutions in San Francisco and situate its development not only within the city's Japanese American communities but also within a shift toward the pan-ethnic Asian American movement.

Tanaka was born in Tokyo in 1943 and in 1967 arrived San Francisco, where he attended the Cherry Blossom Festival, which would become a key site for taiko performance.[33] That festival was the first of a now-annual event in San Francisco's Japantown.[34] The Cherry Blossom Festival was designed to attract new patrons to Japantown's businesses after a redevelopment project, and as ethnomusicologist Benjamin Pachter points out, likely did not resemble the long-running cultural celebrations Tanaka probably experienced as a boy in Japan.[35] Following his disappointment at not hearing drums at the festival (as he had at festivals in Japan), Tanaka began playing taiko in a local Kabuki theater along with other Japanese and Japanese American men, using drums borrowed from a Buddhist temple. At the 1968 Cherry Blossom Festival, Tanaka and a small group of drummers performed. That year, a number of players began to join him in a loosely structured gathering of drummers.[36] Eventually the group started to call itself San Francisco Taiko Dojo, having begun with the less-formal San Francisco Taiko Doukoukai, which, as Pachter points out, aligns it with the loosely affiliated clubs that were common among Japanese American communities in U.S. cities.[37] The term "doukoukai," Pachter notes, reflects the fact that the membership of the group at that time consisted largely of "Japanese immigrants with Japanese as their primary language. It was a gathering point for these immigrants, a way to establish a social circle."[38] The context in which Tanaka began to play taiko, then, was both inspired and supported by Japanese American community institutions: a new community festival, a theater, and a temple.[39]

While San Francisco Taiko Dojo was still in its first year, Kinnara Taiko was formed in Los Angeles in 1969 by members of the Senshin Buddhist Temple. Kinnara Taiko also has a well-rehearsed origin story repeated in documentaries and at taiko events. The young Reverend Masao Kodani had recently begun his leadership at Senshin Buddhist Temple, and one night he and fellow temple member George Abe were putting away the drums the temple used for the annual *obon* festival, the late-summer Japanese festival honoring ancestors, in the summer of 1969 when they began a spontaneous jam session that lasted for hours, until their hands began to bleed. Afterwards, sweating but energized, they looked at each other and decided they should continue to play. As Kodani remembers it, he looked at Abe and said, "George, I think we should do something about this!"[40] The story offers an originary moment for North American taiko that is both spontaneous and rooted in a site of Japanese American community, the Buddhist temple. This story emphasizes spontaneity and serendipity, but Kinnara's development, like San Francisco Taiko Dojo's, was also bolstered by Japanese American institutions and Asian American networks that included young Japanese Americans associated with the temple, the nearby Amerasia bookstore, the radical magazine *Gidra*, and other political and cultural activities. Life history interviews with current and former Kinnara members bear out the trends that placed Japanese Americans and African Americans in geographical—and thus political—proximity to one another, as well as the larger trend of Asian Americans engaging in both radical politics and identity formation described above.[41]

When a curator of the Japanese American National Museum, Sojin Kim, interviewed Masao Kodani for the exhibit *Big Drum: Taiko in the U.S.*, she pressed repeatedly for details beyond the familiar story of the group's origins.[42] Kodani eventually explained that the temple had one drum that was kept in storage year-round, except when played by a single drummer for the obon celebration. The drummer would typically keep the rhythm for the *bon odori* (or obon dancing) that is a central part of the festival. George Abe, who had been involved in a number of Asian American movement efforts, had been learning from the obon drummer, Mr. Inouye.[43] Kodani and Abe had their late-night jam session and were very excited afterward about playing taiko. Abe recalled, "I do remember my hands getting bloody, blisters breaking and just feeling tremendous—this energized kind of feeling from playing that drum." They decided to put together a group and start playing more often.

Kinnara Taiko emerged at Senshin at a moment in the late 1960s when Buddhist temples in the United States were beginning to embrace Japanese arts again after a strong push toward Americanization during World War II. Japanese performing arts, including poetry, music, and theater, had been part of a Buddhist practice known as *horaku*, entertainment designed to teach Buddhist principles, since the arrival of the first Japanese immigrants. The practice, which thrived in the 1920s and 1930s, waned after the war when an emphasis on the English language and assimilation took precedence.[44] Kodani, who came to Senshin in 1968, is credited by many with reviving horaku and for introducing taiko into the repertoire. Kodani characterizes taiko's incorporation into temple activities as largely accidental. It "actually started out as a Buddhist study group," he says, part of a series of retreats that were separate from, but related to, the temple. "So it started off first with chanting and *gagaku* and *bugaku*. And then the taiko thing accident happened and that became fairly big. But . . . there was already a precedent for it here."[45]

Kinnara's first performance in front of an audience was for temple members, and the group soon began playing taiko annually at obon—not as solo drum accompaniment to the dancing, per tradition, but as a group of drummers. Although San Francisco Taiko Dojo had come into being the previous year, the members of Kinnara Taiko had not seen them or anyone else play taiko live in ensemble form before. They learned their *kata*, or form, not from a teacher but from watching a scene in a 1958 Japanese film called *Rickshaw Man* (*Muhomatsu no Issho*, or *"The Life of Wild Matsu"*). In the scene, the leading man, Matsu, attends a festival parade. Seeing a large taiko on one of the floats, he climbs onto it and begins to drum passionately. As his drumming grows wilder, he begins to shed his clothing until he is bare-chested and sweating. It is no surprise that a scene depicting a Japanese man's joyful abandon in the midst of an otherwise staid cultural event served as an inspiration to young sansei taiko drummers who wanted to connect with a wilder side of being Japanese than they typically saw their nisei parents express. In her interview, Sojin Kim inquired of Kodani whether the group simply watched the movie to figure out how to move, and Kodani replied, "Yeah, it was all made up. There was nothing traditional about it at all." Kinnara members, perhaps naively, invented their own taiko tradition after seeing *Rickshaw Man* and accessing their temple drum, but the group's origins also emerge from within the institution of Japanese American Buddhism.[46]

Taiko may have begun during the Asian American movement, but its momentum picked up, rather than faded, as the headier activism of the movement itself waned in the late 1970s. Japanese American community structures—most notably Buddhist churches and temples—continued to support taiko's growth in the United States throughout the 1970s. San Jose Taiko was founded in 1973 at the San Jose Buddhist Temple and later evolved into a performing group inspired by the movement's egalitarian impulses (see Chapter 2). In 1977 taiko began to spread eastward. Denver Taiko, the first group to be formed outside California, was begun by people connected to the Senshin Buddhist Temple in Los Angeles and thus was part of the Japanese American Buddhist taiko movement that Kinnara set off. The Midwest Buddhist Temple in Chicago began using taiko as part of its programming in 1977. And in 1979 Asian Americans in New York decided to start their own group, Soh Daiko. Other groups emerged in California in that decade, as well. In 1976 Stanley Morgan was possibly the first non–Japanese American to start a taiko group in the United States, and Etsuo Hongo, also shin-issei, founded

Los Angeles Matsuri Taiko in 1977.[47] With performances by San Jose Taiko and the Japanese touring group Ondekoza as its inspiration, Katari Taiko of Vancouver, British Columbia, became the first Canadian taiko group in 1979.

Taiko in North America grew significantly in the 1980s and 1990s, with new groups forming in California, Hawaii, and the Pacific Northwest, as well as on the East Coast, in the Midwest, and in the central and eastern areas of Canada. Included in this wave are Kogen Taiko and Mu Daiko, both of which were formed in the Twin Cities of Minneapolis and St. Paul. Kogen Taiko was affiliated with the Midwest Buddhist Temple in Chicago, whereas Mu Daiko was formed as part of a fledgling Asian American theater company, Theater Mu (see Chapter 3). The landscape of Asian America, too, expanded and changed during this time, due in large part to shifts in immigration patterns that occurred after passage of the 1965 Immigration Act. The lifting of bans on immigration from Asia resulted in a much larger, more diverse, and more diffuse population—that is, Asian America was no longer situated only in ethnic enclaves on the coasts but spread throughout the country. Growing gaps in economic status among Asian Americans, as well as in political and ideological outlooks, further challenged the definition of "Asian American community."[48]

The 1990s also saw the development of collegiate taiko groups. The first, Stanford Taiko, emerged when students Ann Ishimaru and Valerie Mih, inspired by a class about taiko and its connections to the Japanese American experience, used student research funds to build a drum and bring in a guest artist for a workshop. This group was followed by several others across the country, and by 2017 there were about 40 collegiate taiko groups, with the concomitant festivals and conferences.[49] Collegiate taiko deserves scholarly attention not only for its huge impact on North American taiko writ large but also for what it might reveal about issues relevant to higher education and Asian America, especially class, access, and racialization.

In recent decades, increasing attention has been given to the transnational and global nature of Asian American communities and identity formation, further complicating the relation between "Asia" and "America."[50] For many groups and individual players, taiko is a transnational practice. Beginning in the 1980s, Kenny and Chizuko Endo spent ten years in Japan studying taiko and other art forms, and San Jose Taiko developed lasting connections with Kodo, one of Japan's best-known touring groups. Tiffany Tamaribuchi spent several years training and touring with Ondekoza in Japan in the late 1990s and continues to collaborate with Japanese artists while running Sacramento Taiko Dan and Jodaiko (see Chapter 5). These are a few representative examples among many other transnational collaborations, tours, and opportunities for study that inform taiko.

The extraordinary growth of taiko during its short time in North America makes it both challenging and rewarding to write about. In the interest of brevity and focus, I am leaving out a number of developments worthy of study, including a host of cross-cultural and cross-genre collaborations, the development of taiko in Hawai'i, and the phenomenon (touched on only briefly in this book) of the impact of the Japanese Exchange and Teaching Programme and other teaching programs.

Beyond these recent developments, the early years of taiko in North America have yet to be documented in detail, and historical analysis of the first ten years of taiko would bring nuance to these histories, which often are simplified and mythologized in the oral tradition. The project of this book, though, is to demonstrate through a close analysis how taiko performs Asian America in multiple historical, geographic, and community contexts.

PERFORMING ASIAN AMERICA

Performance invites questions of identity and collectivity. It is grounded in materiality, produced as it is by and from embodied, historical, and economic circumstances. And yet performance destabilizes the supposed certainties of identity, even ones that are often thought of as unchangeable: race, gender, sexuality, and ability, to name a few. Theatrical performance demonstrates this destabilizing effect in the most obvious ways because actors play roles in which they pretend to be people other than themselves. Thus, as Karen Shimakawa posits, theater "depends on and exposes the fragility of identity (sexed/gendered, racialized, and national) and the complex, dynamic relations between subjects, objects, and the abject."[51] Other forms of performance imperil certainties about identity, too. Josh Kun contends that "[a]ll musical listening is a form of confrontation, of the meeting of worlds and meanings, when identity is made self-aware and is, therefore, menaced through its own interrogation."[52] Throughout the book I invoke the reflections of taiko players (including myself) on the ways taiko prompts awareness and interrogation of multiple and overlapping identities, both individual and collective.

Drumming Asian America asks how people from a range of identity positions, including Asian Americans and Asian Canadians, white and black taiko players, and audiences, co-constitute Asian America through performance. In arguing that North American taiko "drums," or performs, Asian America, this book conceives of it not as a monolithic, unchanging category but as a historically produced and unstable racial formation that is continually being made and remade through policy, immigration, and activism, as well as performance. On the other hand, Asian America is not simply constructed or without material consequence, but, rather, it brings together a set of communities, ideals, actions, contradictions, and debates, and it is put into play not only by Americans of Asian descent but also by policy and media, as well as performers and audiences who may not be Asian American.[53]

I contend that North American taiko performs Asian America, but I am not interested in defining or reifying a category of Asian American performance (or music or dance). Rather, like Deborah Wong, whose approach in *Speak It Louder* shifts from "categories to processes" by focusing on "Asian Americans making music," and Grace Wang, whose study *Soundtracks of Asian America* examines the ways music making shapes Asian Americans' lives, this book focuses on what taiko means to its practitioners and what their embodiments of the form can teach us about Asian America writ large.[54] This shift in ethnomusicology allows scholars to think more broadly about music, in line with Christopher Small's concept of "musicking," which is meant to unburden musical criticism from its fetishization of the text or musical score. Like Richard Schechner's definition of the performance process as extending from the conception and rehearsal stages to the "aftermath" of the performance event, "musicking" is a term that includes any aspect of taking part in making music, from composing to performing or simply listening, even half-consciously, thereby shifting the focus from the art object to acts of taking part in musical performance.[55] Put simply, I am interested in the processes of participating in performance and in examining how performance constitutes Asian America, it-self something that is not static, but put into practice through repeated actions.[56]

The question of what the term "Asian American" means is complex, and as Deborah Wong writes, "part of the discomfort of the question lies in mainstream discomfort over what Asian Americans are."[57] Scholarship on this topic has long rehearsed the notion that Asian America resists definition and is instead constituted by its ever-shifting parameters due to immigration patterns and economic status, by hybridity and complexity among Asian Americans, and by its relation to Americanness.[58] Taiko players negotiate these complexities, too, as they invest in taiko as Japanese, as Japanese American, and as pan-Asian or world music. As Grace Wang writes, "as an organizing principle, a coalition identity, an imagined collectivity, an emerging market segment, a transnational formation, and a census term, the conceptual coherence of the term *Asian American* continually fractures under the weight of its heterogeneity."[59] My project in this book is not to make Asian America cohere but, rather, to understand how taiko points to a range of ideas of what Asian America is. That is, I interrogate the multiple and changing meanings of this concept as it materializes in performances, on stage and off.

As a framework, then, Asian Americanist critique can home in on issues of visibility, foreignness, and coalition, as well as experiences of inclusion, exclusion, and in-betweenness. For North American taiko, such critique can shed light on the investments that players have made in Asian American communities and identities, but also may be useful, as Yutian Wong writes, for "understanding the refusals of Asian Americanness in favor of long-distance belongings to countries outside of the United States, or a desire for a borderless universal subjectivity."[60] When North American taiko players affiliate themselves with taiko as a Japanese or universal art form rather than an Asian American one, whose labor and bodies disappear from view?

Centering the body in studies of performance is a particularly important project for Asian American performance, Yutian Wong argues, since "Asian American performers work in a cultural environment that still finds it difficult to 'see' Asian bodies outside narrow stereotypes—one of which is absence."[61] That is, in the American imagination, Asian Americans are seldom apprehended as performers outside the realm of Western classical music.[62] My work thus focuses not only on performers' words and perspectives but also on the corporeality of taiko performance, how players move—what Matthew Rahaim calls the "musicking body"—and how those movements make meaning for players and audiences.[63] Focusing on bodies calls forth a host of other corporeal, identitarian, and critical concerns that I refer to as cultural politics. My investigation of taiko as it performs Asian America intersects with race, gender, and sexuality, understanding each of these vectors as both lived experience and as called into being through performance.

SEEING WOMEN'S WORK, SOUNDING QUEER POLITICS

In the opening session of the 2015 North American Taiko Conference in Las Vegas, Nevada, longtime taiko community leader Alan Okada stopped abruptly partway through his lecture on the history of North American taiko and apologized to the hundreds of taiko players gathered before him. He acknowledged that all of the players he highlighted in his Power Point presentation were men. The crowd murmured. Flustered, Okada said, "As you know, there are a lot of strong, powerful women with bachi [drumsticks] out there." He went on to point out, as an example, that Kenny Endo's school and ensembles could not function without the tireless efforts of his wife and fellow taiko player, Chizuko Endo. In an interview later that year, Okada spoke to me about the presence of women both on stage and behind the scenes and said that, "in the evolution of taiko in North America there have, other than at the very beginning, there have been *mostly* women in taiko." Not as many, he acknowledged, have been in leadership positions.[64] Nonetheless, Okada's presentation was a telling moment in which women did not make it into the official record of taiko history: their pictures were not on the slides, and their names were not attached to the important milestones.[65] Yet women comprise roughly two-thirds of taiko players in the United States and Canada. The omission of women from Okada's history clearly embarrassed him in the moment, but more important, it underscored the urgency of recording women's roles in the history of taiko as it develops. It also demonstrates a need to craft histories that do not depend on a narrow definition of what constitutes leadership.

If Okada's lecture eclipsed women's work in taiko, a session called "Taiko Talks," curated by conference coordinator Elise Fujimoto, let it shine. In a series of four twenty-minute lectures based on a TED Talk format, four presenters—all of them women—shared how they were using taiko to effect material change in their lives and the lives of others. Karen Young, founder of Genki Spark in Boston, spoke about arts and advocacy in her group of Asian American women, which develops "visible leaders both on and off the stage." Members of Genki Spark train as taiko players and as advocates for the arts and for racial, gender, and LGBTQ equality. Iris Shiraishi, who formed ensemble-MA after her many years with Mu Daiko, discussed the ways taiko has shaped her work as a music therapist, citing studies of the benefits of drumming for people's brains and overall health, as well as describing scenarios about working with developmentally disabled and elderly students. In her talk P. J. Hirabayashi, formerly of San Jose Taiko, introduced her new project Taiko Peace, in which she uses performance, including butoh and taiko, to promote unity in line with principles of the Charter for Compassion. She discussed the effects of racism on her self-esteem when she was in high school, her political awakening in college during the U.S. war with Vietnam, and the powerful effects of seeing women performing Japanese music in new ways in the 1970s, both in folk duo Chris and Joanne's rock-and-roll version of the *bon* dance "Tanko Bushi" and in a mother-daughter pair playing taiko with the San Francisco Taiko Dojo.

The fourth and final presenter was Chieko Kojima, a Japanese national who spoke through translator and taiko collaborator Yuta Kato. Kojima is well known for her many years as a performer with Kodo and as a founder of the Japanese folk performance ensemble Hanayui. She described how becoming an artist helped her "escape" the fate of marrying and having babies that was expected of all Japanese women, and also the isolation she felt as the only woman performer in Kodo, a group whose structure dictated that women could dance but not drum. For eight years she continued with Kodo until a period of depression convinced her to take a break. After spending some time studying dance in Bali, she returned to Kodo and created "Hana Hachijo," a performance piece in which she is very much drummer and dancer at once, and she felt happier and able to continue dancing.

These talks highlighted the material, intellectual, and emotional labor these women have invested in taiko, yet they were nowhere mentioned in the history lesson. With the possible exception of Kojima, whose "Hana Hachijo" has brought her recognition as an artist, these kinds of investments do not result in being thought of as taiko stars, even if they earn the respect of peers. Furthermore, the women's talks highlight taiko as a social and political practice, one that can be engaged in activist, medical, geopolitical, and aesthetic realms.

This book privileges women taiko players as interview subjects and gender as a category of analysis. I have chosen to devote time and attention to groups that have been led or deeply influenced by women taiko players. As Alan Okada's apologetic moment at NATC 2015 indicates, the oral tradition of taiko history already rehearses an established narrative that centers men as the most important leaders, composers, and performers, despite the acknowledgment that there are "a lot of strong, powerful women with bachi out there." They are not only out there; they outnumber men two to one. They lead groups, teach classes, compose and choreograph new works, rework traditionally masculine taiko norms, and make their livings as taiko performers. But on a less visible level, they are also sometimes the people whose artistic innovations influence their own and other groups, even when they are not the sensei or leader; they are often the administrative engines of groups, although systemic factors such as child-rearing or other care-taking responsibilities may prevent them from stepping into the spotlight as often as men do. While this study does not focus exclusively on women or women's groups, I have chosen to highlight groups that allow me to interview a significant number of women taiko players so that I can illustrate the kinds of labor women have performed in service of the taiko community and bring attention to the unconscious biases already at play in still-nascent official and unofficial taiko narratives.

In addition to engaging a critical race lens, this study is also driven by feminist and queer impulses. Beyond the selection of interview subjects, this lens also factors in choosing which performances and off-stage scenarios to analyze. As Paul Yoon and Shawn Bender have pointed out, hypermasculinity is often a valued aesthetic in taiko performance in the United States and Japan.[66] Many taiko practitioners have challenged these norms, both by forging new aesthetics and placing women in traditionally masculine roles, but there is still work to do. Chapters 4 and 5, in particular, engage with a range of gender performances available in taiko, and my approach to masculinity emerges through a queer lens, looking at women's reworkings of traditional material and the ways female masculinity hails queer spectators and performers.

In her Taiko Talk at NATC 2015, Chieko Kojima described a particular dance, the "Nishimonai," in which a lone woman walks slowly across the stage, a long kimono restricting her steps and a large-brimmed hat obscuring her face—and thus her identity—from the audience. This dance was one she performed night after night with Kodo, and for her, its bleak loneliness and anonymity crystallized how she felt as part of the group. The night after Kojima delivered this talk she performed at the Taiko Jam, the curated concert that is a highlight of each North American Taiko Conference. Kojima performed "Hana Hachijo," the duet for taiko for which she has become known. The piece typically features two drummers: one, often a man playing a base beat, is mostly obscured behind the drum, which is laid on its side atop a tall stand about shoulder height, and the other, Kojima, dressed in a kimono and positioned in a pool of light (figures 1.2 and 1.3). Although the two drummers' rhythms interlock, the focus remains on Kojima, whose fast sticking creates blurred blooms around her head and torso as she swirls her bachi around her head, under her arms, and off the center and edges of the drum.

For this performance she began in the usual way, alone in the spotlight, beating slowly on the face of the drum. But she was soon joined by a multitude of young drummers, pairs of them placed on the spacious stage, playing alongside her, their sticks swirling—perhaps not quite as agilely as hers—and their knees bending as they moved through the song's light yet grounded choreography. As the piece reached its climax, Kojima left her drum and started dancing on the apron of the stage, smiling and winding through the other drummers. She and the other drummers were together, not alone; her face was open and smiling, not obscured; their energy was buoyant, not somber. During the finale, when all the groups on the program played a final number together, Kojima again danced through the other drummers, throwing colorful confetti (figure 1.4). The moment was pure joy. Sitting in the audience for both the talk and the performance allowed me to see how Kojima had harnessed performance to revisit and repair the pain she had experienced early in her career: she was once a woman alone crossing the stage night after night, alone in a group of male performers, alone as a dancer when she wanted to drum. Here,

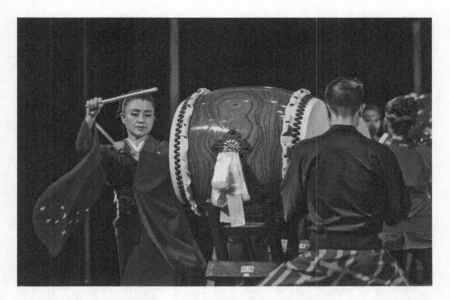

Figure 1.2. Chieko Kojima and Yuta Kato perform "Hana Hachijo" at the 2015 Taiko Jam, Las Vegas, Nevada. Photo by Raymond Yuen, Yuen Designs. Photo courtesy of the Taiko Community Alliance. Used with permission.

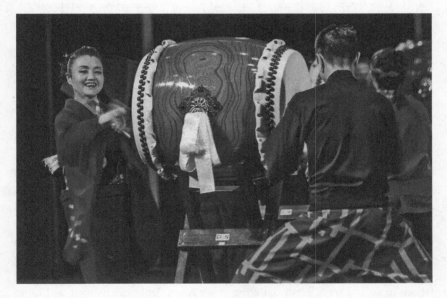

Figure 1.3. Chieko Kojima, Yuta Kato, and members of Unit One perform "Hana Hachijo" at the 2015 Taiko Jam, Las Vegas, Nevada. Photo by Raymond Yuen, Yuen Designs. Photo courtesy of the Taiko Community Alliance. Used with permission.

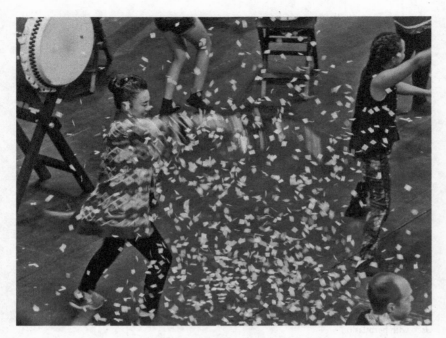

Figure 1.4. Chieko Kojima throws confetti during the finale of the 2015 Taiko Jam, Las Vegas, Nevada. Photo by Gene Sugano. Photo courtesy of the Taiko Community Alliance. Used with permission.

she invited others, women and men, to share her joy in drumming. It was a deeply moving experience to hear the talk and watch the performance, to understand the history and the gendered politics behind her iconic performance piece, and finally to see her wrest her experience into something new that celebrated her freedom to drum and her joy in being together with others onstage.

This joy of being in community extends to queer taiko players as well, and this book attends to the ways sexuality operates in taiko both as a communitarian and an aesthetic concern. Scholarship concerning taiko and sexuality is scarce, but the form's erotic appeal is great. Deborah Wong writes about taiko as a "passionately appealing" practice for Asian American women in its reconfiguration of "women's work," even as taiko performances remain open to Orientalist spectatorship.[67] Paul Yoon's work on taiko and Asian American masculinity in performance acknowledges the possibility of gay male spectatorship in certain taiko performances, but lesbian spectatorship and female masculinity in taiko have yet to be explored.[68] Bringing queer theory and performance studies to bear on taiko opens up the critical terrain in several ways. First, centering queer Asian American women, as I do in Chapter 5, addresses the overwhelming whiteness of queer performance studies and contributes to a growing body of scholarship about queer women and queer people of color. Second, while Asian Americans have been engaged in LGBTQ activism since at least the late 1970s, it is also true that homophobia is an issue within some Asian American communities and within U.S. culture as a whole.[69] Finally, in naming sexuality as a key facet of taiko performance, I not only foreground the presence of queer-identified performers but also highlight the erotic and pleasurable aspects of taiko performance. I, like Ramón Rivera-Servera, approach queerness as both an identity and "a continuous process of becoming" queer through acts both spectacular and mundane.[70] To be an audience member at a taiko performance is often to feel vibrations in your own body, to watch people move and sweat as they labor at the drums, and to hear the resonant sounds of drums and the guttural yells the performers use to mark time and encourage each other onstage. Yet the erotic power of taiko often goes unacknowledged among taiko players and sometimes in taiko scholarship. Applying queer studies frameworks that emphasize sex and sexuality, this work extends Yoon's and Wong's engagement with taiko's erotic appeal.

MOVING THROUGH THE BOOK

The narrative arc that informs the rest of the book begins in 1973 with the formation of San Jose Taiko and concludes with a discussion of taiko and activism in 2017. The chapters overlap chronologically because they are arranged in the order in which the various groups under discussion were formed. I begin, then, in California, home to at least one-half of all North American taiko players, in the 1970s before moving to the Midwest beginning in the late 1990s to examine the shifting landscape of Asian America. The last two chapters, less tied to geography, take a more conceptual approach than the others to consider, first, whiteness, blackness, and gender in the early twenty-first century and then queer theory and Asian Canadian community festivals in Vancouver, where the all-women's group Jodaiko has been performing annually since 2006. This book looks at taiko not only as it appears in fully produced concerts but also in festival contexts, educational outreach performances, and rehearsal spaces.

In the first part of the book I establish connections between the so-called pioneer taiko groups and Asian American movement activism, ties that directly inform San Jose Taiko and indirectly inform Mu Daiko. These two chapters focus on multiple sites of encounter between taiko and audiences and analyze the meanings produced in these on- and offstage scenarios. Chapter 2 establishes the context in which taiko emerged in the United States, specifically California, and argues that San Jose Taiko, via its engagement with Asian American history and its practice of the taiko folk dance "Ei Ja Nai Ka?" in concerts, obon, and taiko gatherings, draws on its activist roots to embody and share Asian American immigrant histories. I discuss the difficulties that San Jose Taiko has in maintaining its identity as an Asian American group in Orientalist performance and marketing contexts that want to see the group as exotic. Chapter 3 moves from the West Coast to the Midwest to broaden the book's conception of Asian American performance, audience expectations, and sites of encounter. The chapter challenges usual conceptions of Minnesota (often imagined as white) and of Asian America (often thought of as concentrated on the coasts) by examining the Minneapolis-based group Mu Daiko. This chapter delves further into themes introduced in Chapter 2, focusing closely on outreach as a scenario of discovery to elucidate the complex and unique Asian American communities in Minnesota, with a focus on adopted Korean American members of Mu Daiko. Taken together, these two chapters make the case that taiko performs Asian America, even as it is practiced by people from a variety of identity positions. They also highlight the ways Asian American activism continues well beyond the late 1960s and early 1970s, in which it has been circumscribed.

The second half of the book brings intersectional analysis into sharper focus by thinking through race, gender, and sexuality together. Chapter 4 opens up the critical lens of *Drumming Asian America* to consider how white and black women perform Asian America through their practice of taiko. This chapter, which extends an autoethnographic approach established in Chapter 3, argues that white women experience and produce ambivalence in taiko performance by unsettling audiences' Orientalist expectations and by negotiating their own, sometimes new racial awareness as taiko performers. Black women's experiences point to the ways they and Asian Americans are triangulated vis-à-vis white people. Chapter 4 ends with the suggestion that taiko offers a potential site for enacting cross-racial intimacies not only through the proximity of white and black women to Asian American co-performers, but through the very alienation and ambivalence that participating in such performance can produce for players who are not Asian American. In a departure from the previous two chapters, which are firmly located in cities, this chapter is located more conceptually than geographically, using a multi-sited ethnographic approach.

The final chapter of the book focuses on the confluence of queerness, gender, and Asian America. Using close performance analysis, as well as ethnographic interviews and autoethnography, Chapter 5 argues that the women's group Jodaiko, led by Tiffany Tamaribuchi, queers North American taiko via performance choices, the gender performances of its members, and the undeniable sensuality and eroticism of live taiko performance. This chapter addresses the homophobia that is still present—despite recent legislative gains—in the United States, in Asian American communities, and in the taiko community. Tiffany Tamaribuchi's pick-up group centers Asian American queer women on stage, producing a visible "homo-geneity" and performing so-called traditional taiko pieces within a queer/butch aesthetic. In the conclusion I locate the first-ever Women and Taiko gathering in San Diego as a site for cross-racial exchange in taiko and consider the role of performance and joy in activism.

This book is deeply informed by my experiences as a practitioner, teacher, and fan of taiko for over eighteen years. I was a taiko player before I was a scholar, and decisions about how to approach this book were made with the knowledge that taiko players will probably read it. Where possible, I invited people I had interviewed to read drafts of the chapters and to engage in dialogue with me about the ideas and arguments they contain. My methods are deeply embodied. Each chapter herein draws on a wide variety of materials and sources, including ethnographic interviews, participant-observation, performance analysis based on live performance and on photo and video documentation, archival materials, and informal interviews and conversations. Between 2009 and 2017 I conducted twenty-five interviews with individual taiko players, and I also conducted a group interview with San Jose Taiko members who were on tour in Austin, Texas, in 2009. The activities I include in the category "participant-observation" span a range of opportunities from attending performances, taking workshops at taiko gatherings, performing alongside those I write about, riding along to performance events, and attending taiko conferences to simply spending time with taiko players, all of this officially beginning in 2009, when I began researching my dissertation, but in reality beginning ten years earlier when I took my first taiko class in Minneapolis. I also draw on Life History Interviews conducted by the Japanese American National Museum staff. Most other materials, besides the occasional newspaper review or commercially or electronically available video documentation, are part of my personal archive. That is, I rely on my embodied knowledge of taiko to re-create in words the kinds of pleasures and challenges taiko presents to its performers. And many of the ideas presented herein stem from ideas that began to form while I was a taiko performer, negotiating on- and offstage interactions, identities, and challenges.

Scholarship moves slowly, and in the time I was researching and writing this book, taiko has grown and changed at a surprisingly fast pace. For some, my focus on the relation between taiko and Asian American cultural politics will seem like a throwback to the bad old days of identity politics. Indeed, in 2013 I gave a presentation as part of a scholarly panel dedicated to taiko at the annual conference of the Society for Ethnomusicology, a panelist expressed frustration with the apparently narrow focus of North American taiko scholarship on issues of identity. At a moment when there had yet to be a single monograph published on North American taiko, let alone a long history of taiko scholarship focusing on Asian American cultural politics, it was premature to call the moment over when it had hardly begun. Still, it is important to acknowledge the contested terrain that taiko occupies for both practitioners and scholars. But rather than accede to a call to move on from taiko scholarship that engages Asian American (or other racial, gender, or sexual) cultural politics, I believe that this is the very moment to elucidate for scholars, for audiences, and, most crucially, for taiko players the Asian American roots of taiko and the ways in which every player's participation contributes to how U.S. audiences see and experience Asian American—and American—cultural politics.

CHAPTER 2
A New Taiko Folk Dance

San Jose Taiko and Asian American Movements

"Dig! And pick! And dig! And pick!" A woman's voice shouts over the din of makeshift taiko drums and excited voices as hundreds of taiko players spill out of the Aratani Japan America Theater in Japantown, Los Angeles. It is nine-thirty at night, a rousing taiko concert has just ended inside the theater, and the audience—mostly participants in the 2009 North American Taiko Conference—has now gathered outside on the one-acre plaza and is ready to dance. Together, we bounce forward and backward in rhythm while rolling our forearms in front of us, we hop on one leg, and we wipe sweat from our brows. These movements are the stylized gestures of "Ei Ja Nai Ka?" (Isn't it good?), a participatory folk dance created by P. J. Hirabayashi that is one of San Jose Taiko's signature works. By digging, picking, and sweating together, we dancers honor the memory and labor of the issei, who were the first generation of Japanese immigrants in the United States. A swingy rhythm from the *chappa*, small hand-held cymbals, cuts through the rumble of plastic garbage-bins-turned-drums keeping the base beat for a widening circle of dancers. Drummers shout, "Ei Ja Nai Ka!" and dancers respond, "A So-re, A So-re!" Then, "Ei Ja Nai Ka, hai!" "A So-re, So-re, Yoi-sho!" This call-and-response pattern continues for a few rounds before the *shinobue* (a bamboo flute) joins in, and voices singing in Japanese float over the din in a melodic song.

It is a hot summer night, and after a few rounds of digging, picking, and jumping my way around the plaza, I step back to watch. The crowd is racially mixed, mostly Asian Americans with many white, as well as a few black and Latino/a men and women. There are people in their twenties, those who are middle-aged, and those with bodies small and large. Some execute the gestures with confidence. Others shuffle through the steps looking confused. There are people who, instead of dancing, loiter at the center of or outside the circle to watch and socialize. For some participants this is their first introduction to this folk dance, while others anticipate dancing "Ei Ja Nai Ka?" in this ritual that takes place after the Saturday night Taiko Jam concert at every North American Taiko Conference. After years of trying to pick it up on the fly at different conferences, I am glad to have finally learned the dance in a workshop with San Jose Taiko members earlier that day. The dance continues for twenty more minutes before the circle begins to break up and the summer sky continues to darken above the downtown lights.[1] Flushed with the joy of dancing, the participants collect their belongings and disperse to the hotels, sushi counters, and karaoke bars of Japantown. This small business district tucked south of U.S. Highway 101 (referred to locally as the 101) in downtown Los Angeles bursts into life during taiko conferences, as hundreds of taiko players patronize businesses selling Japanese pastries, noodles, newspapers, imported knick-knacks, and other goods and services. For some Los Angeles-area taiko players this is home base, a familiar site of many years of civic, political, community, and cultural gatherings, but for many players from across the United States and Canada, these few blocks are as close to Japan as they have ever been. Similarly, for some participants the histories evoked in "Ei Ja Nai Ka?" are familiar, and for others it is an embodied introduction to the early history of Japanese immigration.

Hirabayashi's "Ei Ja Nai Ka?" is a taiko and dance piece that San Jose Taiko teaches widely in workshops and at festivals.[2] It is different from most taiko songs, in which drummers' movements stem from striking the drum, rather than dancing separately. San Jose Taiko describes the piece as a "taiko folk dance," situating the work within taiko musical repertory and other participatory group dances performed at obon festivals, cherry blossom festivals, and other Japanese American community celebrations.[3] The use of "folk" signals both its demonstration of ethnic roots and its participatory nature. The Saturday night Taiko Jam concert is the pièce de résistance of the biennial North American Taiko Conference, an opportunity for attendees to see a carefully curated lineup of four taiko groups. It is a tradition for the audience—largely comprised of taiko players—to erupt into the now-expected, but seemingly spontaneous, performance of "Ei Ja Nai Ka?" immediately after the Taiko Jam. Many taiko players learn the song, as I did, during a workshop at the conference.[4] Non-taiko players might learn the dance part as well, if they happen to see San Jose Taiko perform at an obon festival or in another community setting that encourages audience participation. The piece is intentionally participatory. The choreography is simple and the musical composition is catchy enough to encourage audiences to embody its rhythms and gestures by joining the circle of dancers. Much taiko repertoire, including other San Jose Taiko pieces, emphasizes technical prowess, group cohesion, and rhythmic complexity. But with its relative simplicity, "Ei Ja Nai Ka?" closes the gap between audience and performers, blurring the boundaries between the two. Participants who are just learning can dance and chant alongside seasoned San Jose Taiko members. Even as a novice at the dance steps, I was at once performer and spectator.

This chapter makes explicit connections between taiko and cultural politics by focusing on how the politics of the Asian American movement inspired and continue to resonate within the performances and practices of San Jose Taiko. The phrase "Asian American Movements" in the title refers to both the embodied and choreographed aspects of taiko performance and the constellation of political activities undertaken by Asian American activists beginning in the late 1960s. In order to explore the intertwined relation between these two meanings of "movement," this chapter undertakes three readings of San Jose Taiko's work. Before launching into the analyses, I first establish the historical and theoretical frameworks of the chapter. Then, in my first reading, I situate San Jose Taiko within a genealogy of North American taiko and within the emergence of Asian American identity and politics. This contextualizes the group's effort to develop an Asian American sensibility in the face of external demands for Japanese authenticity as a complex navigation of aesthetic and sociopolitical terrain. Second, I analyze "Ei Ja Nai Ka?" as a tribute to issei labor and pre-internment history. In performing and sharing this work, San Jose Taiko reflects movement-era values of developing an Asian American consciousness and creating grass-roots, revisionist Japanese American histories. With its specific focus on the issei, the first Japanese immigrants to the United States, "Ei Ja Nai Ka?" demonstrates San Jose Taiko's commitment to taiko as an Asian American art form and suggests ways for those who are not Asian American to participate in and co-construct "Asian America" through participatory performance. Finally, I offer an analysis of marketing materials from San Jose Taiko's 2009 national tour to highlight how the group attempts to remain grounded in Asian America when presenters and advertisers frame their performances as exotic and foreign.

SAN JOSE TAIKO IN CONTEXT

The members of San Jose Taiko have long held leadership positions among North American taiko players and in particular at the North American Taiko Conference (NATC) and regional taiko gatherings. As the 2016 Taiko Census results show, Asian Americans still comprise the largest percentage of taiko players, but approximately 40 percent of survey participants do not identify themselves as Asian American.[5] As the taiko community expands and its practitioners come to taiko via avenues not linked to Japanese American or Asian American cultural contexts, the tradition of dancing "Ei Ja Nai Ka?" can be seen as a way to remind taiko players of the form's genealogy in the United States, which is inextricably linked to Asian American history and cultural politics.

The founding members of San Jose Taiko, which was formed in 1973, describe their involvement in Asian American movement (AAM) activities as connected to their taiko activities.[6] This movement, influenced by the civil rights movement, the black power movement, and global Third World activism, brought together Asians of different ethnic backgrounds to fight for broad-based social change. The AAM encompassed ethnic consciousness-raising efforts as well as antiwar demonstrations, education reform, and grassroots activities focused on helping underserved communities.[7] For the most part, Japanese Americans involved in the movement were sansei, or third-generation, although some younger nisei (second-generation) were also involved.[8] In his book *The Asian American Movement* historian William Wei contends that the AAM began to wind down in the early 1970s, but more recent scholarship by Micheal Liu, Kim Geron, and Tracy Lai argues that AAM activities extended beyond the early 1970s and that movement participants continue to be community leaders who make significant change within and beyond Asian American communities.[9] Although the height of its activism took place in the late 1960s and early 1970s, the AAM has had a lasting impact on the participants who continued their work. The formation of San Jose Taiko was a result of movement activism, and situating taiko within the narrative of the AAM foregrounds the role of performance in enacting the movement's ideals and in political protest more generally. Many of the ideals that San Jose Taiko embraced were informed by the movement; these include negotiating identity-related issues as well as the instantiation of practices that reflect "peace, social justice, and equality."[10] These ideals are reflected in the choice to honor early immigrant labor in their performances.

When San Jose Taiko members perform "Ei Ja Nai Ka?" at concerts, festivals, and other community gatherings, they stage a history of Japanese American immigrant labor. Hirabayashi dedicates the song to the issei and "celebrates Japanese American history through movements that reflect the Issei's work in agriculture, mining, and railroad construction."[11] The piece "re-members" (to borrow a phrase from Ngugi wa Thiong'o) Japanese American history in that it both enacts social memory and re-embodies that history in the present.[12] This re-membering in dance and music has historiographic implications. Theater historian Charlotte Canning argues for performance as a viable means of conveying history: performance "can encourage considerations of the gestural, the emotional, the aural, the visual, and the physical in ways beyond print's ability to evoke or understand them."[13] "Ei Ja Nai Ka?" connects its performers and spectators—some the grandchildren or great-grandchildren of the issei about whom the song was written, some newcomers to Japanese American history—to "the past" using the gestural life of manual labor. The piece "actively place[s] the past in the community context of the present time" through a complex interplay of dancing, drumming, singing, and chanting.[14] "Ei Ja Nai Ka?" articulates issei history in ways beyond those available in narrative histories. Within the layers of music and dance, and within the various contexts in which the piece is offered, the dance evokes pre-internment labor and immigration, aspects of Japanese American history often overshadowed by the intense focus on incarceration. It is important to acknowledge that internment is one traumatic event in the longer narrative of Japanese American history, which encompasses exploitative labor conditions, racist property laws, and other injustices, many of which reflect ongoing issues related to U.S. immigration policy.

DOING AUTHENTICITY, NAVIGATING ASIAN AMERICA

San Jose Taiko has become one of the most recognized and respected North American taiko ensembles and was the third taiko group in the United States. Like its predecessors San Francisco Taiko Dojo and Kinnara Taiko, the group is linked to a local Japanese American institution. Its founders, Roy Hirabayashi, Reverend Hiroshi Abiko, and Dean Miyakusu, were interested in drawing youth to the San Jose Buddhist Temple by hosting "cool" activities.[15] The group continues to foster strong ties to local Japanese American institutions while maintaining a touring schedule that takes them across the United States and abroad. Among other awards, in 2011 the National Endowment for the Arts recognized founding members and former directors P. J. and Roy Hirabayashi with a National Heritage Fellowship, a prestigious award that celebrates the recipients' artistry and acknowledges their craft as of national importance.[16] The pair, a married couple, has bequeathed their roles as artistic director and executive director to longtime group members Franco Imperial and Wisa Uemura, but they continue to be involved with the group and to offer artistic and leadership-focused workshops and mentorship to taiko groups internationally.

San Jose Taiko was inspired and guided in its formative years by San Francisco Taiko Dojo and Kinnara Taiko, and later by several Japanese taiko groups formed in the late 1960s. Several of San Jose Taiko's early members were involved in the Asian American movement, including antiwar activism, community service projects, and the formation of ethnic studies programs in California colleges. The group's philosophy was shaped to a large extent by the AAM's critique of oppressive structures. Today, in keeping with San Jose Taiko's activist roots, as new members join, regardless of their racial or ethnic identity, they are expected to learn about Asian American history and the yellow power movement, another way of describing the Asian American movement that emphasizes its connections to the black power movement. The group operates in an egalitarian manner with a consensus-based structure. San Jose Taiko's membership is open to people of any gender, race, or ethnicity; and although membership has consistently been comprised mainly of Asian Americans, the group has included a number of non-Asian members throughout its history.

On stage, the group (pictured in figure 2.1) exudes a cohesion that exceeds its technical precision as the performers communicate through glances, smiles, yells, and the ever-present bouncy pulse that seems to rise up from their feet, through torsos and arms, and into the drums. As one reviewer noted, San Jose Taiko's drummers are "not only one with their instruments, but with each other."[17] With

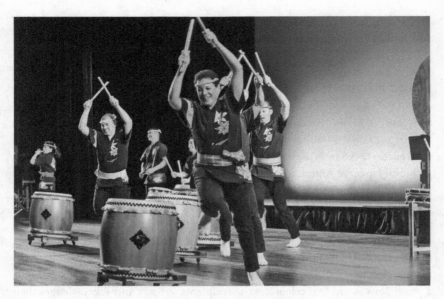

Figure 2.1. San Jose Taiko members in concert, 2013. www.taiko.org. Photo by Higashi Design. Used with permission.

few solo and duet numbers, their concerts emphasize ensemble work. The players move together with a light yet grounded energy. Ethnomusicologist Deborah Wong writes of the "exuberance and joy" she feels while watching them: "They have this fantastic energy, and it's different from any other taiko group. Their technique and their level of skill is very high—enviably so—but you can also see the community base in their playing. Or maybe I just think I see it because I *know* it's there: I know several of their members and I've seen how they interact with other taiko players."[18] San Jose Taiko has strong ties not only to other taiko players, but also to San Jose's Japantown, particularly its annual obon festival, at which they regularly perform "Ei Ja Nai Ka?"

As the group formed its aesthetic and philosophical style during its early years, members grappled with competing and overlapping notions of Japaneseness, authenticity, and Asian American identity.[19] As they sought training from other groups, San Jose Taiko contended with how to maintain cultural authenticity vis-à-vis Japanese customs, while also remaining true to their members' political beliefs. Many of the Japanese Americans who began playing taiko in the 1970s found it appealing because it was both associated with Japan—and therefore a way to connect with their cultural roots and the issei—and a powerful and engaging art form that countered prevailing images of Japanese Americans as quiet and passive. Interviews with taiko players from this period reveal that for many, other traditional Japanese arts such as ikebana, or flower arranging, and traditional dance were not considered powerful (likely because they are coded as feminine) but rather delicate and meditative—exactly how they did not want to be perceived in the 1970s.

Although taiko served these two distinct purposes, they did not always mesh. Some of the Japanese customs that San Jose Taiko was encouraged to adopt went against the grain of their ethics, particularly regarding oppressive hierarchies and gender equality issues.

When San Jose Taiko formed in 1973, they were a small but dedicated group of Asian Americans—activists, students, and music aficionados—who had bought a thousand dollars' worth of drums from the fledgling Kinnara Taiko and who made up their own rhythms in the basement of the San Jose Buddhist Temple because they believed that taiko gave expression to their experiences as Asians in America. A black-and-white photograph of a 1979 informal gathering shows seven young shaggy-haired Asian American men and women standing behind their drums in a paved courtyard. It is a candid snapshot, taken during a jam session (see figure 2.2). Whereas in a more formal setting they might have worn happi coats (short, colorful coats), *tabi* (split-toed footwear), and *hachimaki* (headbands), here the puffy jackets, bell-bottom jeans, and feathered hair situate the group squarely in the 1970s, part of the counterculture.

Early San Jose Taiko members were largely improvising this newly adopted art form, as were Kinnara and San Francisco Taiko Dojo, but they nonetheless experienced taiko as a material connection to Japanese diasporic culture, a relationship they would continue to negotiate throughout the group's history. Returning to the idea of musicking, shifting focus from the art object to the acts of taking part in musical performance, helps reveal how San Jose Taiko grappled with issues of identity

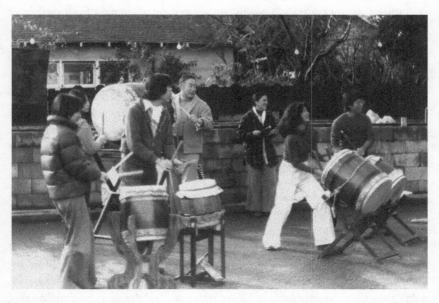

Figure 2.2. San Jose Taiko pioneers in outdoor rehearsal, 1979. Roy Hirabayashi plays small *sumo* drum, third from left, and P. J. Hirabayashi plays the *atarigane*, fifth from left. www.taiko.org. Photo courtesy of the San Jose Taiko Conservatory Archive. Used with permission.

as it created its own style and repertoire.[20] This shift from performance object and text to the acts of making music also opens up an important shift to the bodies that participate in performance as players and audience members. This chapter focuses not only on the performers' choices but also on the corporeality of taiko performance and how players move—what Matthew Rahaim calls the "musicking body."[21] Small writes that "performance does not exist in order to present musical works, but rather, musical works exist in order to give performers something to perform."[22] For example, current executive director Wisa Uemura emphasizes that San Jose Taiko made a conscious choice to compose new music, rather than learn any existing Japanese repertoire, because "the charter members were not as familiar with Japanese music stylings (taiko or not) and they wanted music that represented them as Japanese-Americans."[23] Taiko materialized through situated experiences of Japanese Americans and Asian Americans, including the music styles that already resided in their bodies.

Like many performers working in neofolk or invented traditions, San Jose Taiko players grappled with notions of being authentically Japanese while also embracing taiko's relative newness. Looking at taiko as musicking—as a "doing and a thing done," to borrow Elin Diamond's notion of performance—positions taiko as a space for doing or performing authenticity, rather than succumbing to a notion of authenticity as a stable or static state of being.[24] As historian Gary Okihiro writes, "Like all identities, although but a script, Japanese gains form and currency through theory and practice."[25] That is, identities such as Japanese and Asian American are called into being, in part, through repeated performances, through rehearsal.

Rather than measure itself against an elusive yet seemingly fixed quality of Japaneseness, San Jose Taiko sought to create an authentic, pan-ethnic Asian American practice. Looking back on the group's early years, Roy Hirabayashi said, "Well, naturally, when we first started, there was no real *kata* [form] for us. There [were] no costumes. Our look was Kikkoman Shoyu happi coats with bellbottom pants and long hair."[26] Most likely referring to Seiichi Tanaka and San Francisco Taiko Dojo, Roy recalled, "We got in trouble early on because people, the traditionalists, were complaining that you can't use a tambourine with taiko or a cowbell. That's not taiko." San Jose's early attempts to incorporate non-Japanese instruments into its practice met with criticism, but those innovations are now commonplace in many taiko groups.

Although many American taiko players see Japanese taiko as authentic, the Japanese tradition, too, is comprised of multiple influences, including American jazz.[27] Even if authenticity is an elusive goal, it nonetheless circulates as an important concept in taiko circles. In an interview with the Japanese American National Museum, P. J. Hirabayashi describes the conundrum of attempting to achieve authenticity in a diasporic form: "We'll never be Japanese from Japan because we didn't grow up in the environment." She continues, "And therefore, you could never play Japanese taiko like Japanese taiko. So we have to be very realistic that what we play is definitely from our experiences."[28] Performance theorist Joni L. Jones writes that although it is tempting to eschew authenticity as hopelessly essentialist, such a viewpoint "disregard[s] the passionate longing that undergirds the hope of authenticity." Jones offers a definition of authenticity as something one does rather than something one finds. Performance allows a person to embody aspects of culture, creating a "new authenticity, based on body knowledge, on what audiences and performers share together, on what they mutually construct."[29] Jones's formulation acknowledges performance as a site that is constituted by performers' choices and audience members' responses. What did San Jose Taiko want to co-construct with its audiences?

Rather than imitate Japanese taiko, San Jose Taiko consciously constructed itself as Asian American. In a move that distinguished them from San Francisco Taiko Dojo, whose leader Seiichi Tanaka's way of doing authenticity relied on his direct connections to Japan, San Jose Taiko created new music and practices that reflected their members' identities. Realizing that they could not be "Japanese from Japan," the members of San Jose Taiko reframed their endeavor as an authentically Asian American taiko group, one that was inspired by their experiences as community activists, their multiethnic membership, and their eclectic musical tastes. Although they adopted some of Tanaka's practices, their choosing the term "Asian American taiko" was in part a way to forge their own practice, based on their own experiences as Asians in the United States. This was not a move away from Japanese taiko—the group has maintained strong connections to many Japanese groups—but rather a way to purposefully embrace a multiply influenced form that drew inspiration from members' musical tastes, including American vernacular music and Afro-Cuban rhythms.

San Jose Taiko members' desires for a connection to Japan were also mediated through AAM-related activities and ideology. In particular, the U.S. war in Vietnam gave rise to a burgeoning ethnic consciousness among young Asian Americans in the late 1960s and early 1970s.[30] Longtime member P. J. Hirabayashi described how antiwar protests shaped her racial awareness and led her to see herself as an Asian American, rather than as a "progressive, white, anti-war" college student. As she, like many Asian Americans, began to believe that the United States was fighting a racist war in Asia, she also "really became aware of the social injustices within America."[31] Hirabayashi was one of many Asian American students at Berkeley to become politicized during the late 1960s.

In addition to identity-related issues, San Jose Taiko's involvement in the Asian American movement created an impetus toward structural change. Over the course of many years, the group committed itself to creating a collective organizational structure in which all of its members operate as equals. The principle of equality outweighed adherence to what many perceive as a Japanese tradition of organizational structure in which members are ranked according to seniority and defer to those above them in the hierarchy. Hirabayashi believes that hierarchies create oppressive structures in groups. She began to recognize that "just because it's Japanese, you don't have to embrace it . . . if it's something that's oppressive, don't embrace it. That was very conscious."[32] Although San Jose Taiko learned technique and performance skills from Tanaka, they chose not to embrace his group's seniority-based hierarchy, referred to in Japanese as the *sempai-kohai* system. Their decision to treat all members as equals and to reject the oppressive hierarchies of Japanese taiko also meant that women participate as equals, rather than re-creating gendered patterns of behavior, as was the case not only in San Francisco Taiko Dojo (a topic I discuss further in Chapter 5) but also within the AAM and other New Left movements.[33]

Decisions are made by consensus, and all members share responsibility for the group's operations, from costume making and maintaining the rehearsal space to teaching classes and mentoring new members. Although several members hold paid administrative and artistic positions, San Jose Taiko purposefully encourages all members to serve as leaders—and followers—in a variety of capacities. The members learned from Kinnara Taiko and others how to make their own drums from wine barrels, and today the entire group shares the task of creating and maintaining the drums and other instruments they play.[34] In some taiko groups men and women wear slightly different costumes, while in others the sensei wears a special happi coat indicating leadership status. All San Jose Taiko members, including P. J. and Roy, wear exactly the same costume, without any visual markers of seniority or skill. The group also requires an intensive training program that allows all members to play any part in the repertoire, so all have opportunities to play the most desirable or challenging parts. This not only engenders a uniform movement style on stage but also discourages any member from becoming the virtuoso or star.

In large part by necessity, San Jose Taiko members began to compose their own songs early on, fitting the rhythms of their musical influences into the form and movement style they'd learned from their mentors. In the early 1980s, for example, P. J. Hirabayashi created a new taiko composition that was based on a Japanese style of drumming and dancing but pulled its content from the experiences of the issei.

LABORED GESTURES, PERFORMING RACIAL PROGRESS

When San Jose Taiko performs and teaches "Ei Ja Nai Ka?" at festivals, concerts, or taiko gatherings, it connects its artistic work to its AAM and community roots. It also makes explicit how taiko bridged a generational gap between the issei and sansei generations. The piece highlights the issei experience, as did historian Yuji Ichioka, as a "labor history."[35] The first three U.S. taiko groups are often referred to as the pioneer groups;[36] pioneering not only evokes the American frontier but also rhetorically connects these sansei-led groups with issei historians, who cast the first generation as pioneers with a legitimate stake in American "frontier expansionism" in the early twentieth century.[37] Not only did San Jose Taiko's early members and other sansei respect the "adventurous" spirit of the Issei, but sansei in many cities started social service organizations dedicated to caring for the issei—and later generations—as they aged.[38] Sansei, especially those who had become politicized during the Asian American movement, diverged from what they saw as the nisei generation's "accommodationist and assimilationist" political strategies.[39] Many in the nisei generation came of age during the World War II era and lived through the experience of internment. The fear of persecution before, during, and after internment explains, in part, the difference between the nisei generation's more cautious political stances and the more radical activism undertaken by many sansei.[40] The political climate in the United States at mid-century reinforced the nisei tendency toward assimilationist politics. Many avenues of political maneuvering had been foreclosed to them because of a number of sociopolitical pressures during the early twentieth century. The Great Depression, the troubled relations between Japan and the United States leading to World War II, domestic racism, and wartime internment all compelled nisei toward assimilationist politics and away from "affirm[ing] their ethnicity and practic[ing] ethnic politics."[41] Thus, some sansei not only practiced more radical politics than their Nisei parents did but also sought cultural avenues for exploring their Japaneseness.[42]

The sansei push to reclaim their Japanese heritage was informed by a complex dynamic of domestic racism, ethnic pride, and radical AAM politics. Sansei taiko players saw the issei generation as their link to Japanese heritage. Many sansei connected directly with issei through community activism including social services (a branch of AAM embraced by other Asian American communities as well). Others made this connection via the arts, and taiko was one avenue for doing so. After performing taiko at an issei picnic in the late 1970s, P. J. Hirabayashi recalled that many of the audience members were very moved and told San Jose Taiko members, "'Oh, I'm so happy that you are being in touch with your Japanese culture. It makes me very proud.'" She continued, "And to hear that made it sound like it's coming from my grandmother."[43] Though taiko was a recently developed folk art form, the issei recognized and appreciated sansei efforts to embrace Japanese culture via this new tradition. For sansei the sense of connection with Japan was deeply felt, and taiko (albeit a hybrid in many ways) became a means of connecting with issei, many of whom could not speak English. Thus, sansei embraced taiko as a new Japanese American cultural practice produced by historical circumstances that created markedly different experiences for issei, nisei, and sansei.

San Jose Taiko specifically honors the connection between the issei and sansei in "Ei Ja Nai Ka?" through gesture and lyrics. Creator P. J. Hirabayashi notes that she was inspired by specific Japanese folk traditions and ensembles, tying the piece in aesthetic terms to Japanese performance. The gestural movements used in the piece mimic the movements of labor performed by issei—and, by extension, other immigrants and exploited populations—in their first years in the United States. Group members explain that the rough translation of the title, "Isn't it good?," implies an acknowledgment of the good things among the bad and a recognition of the sacrifices that have contributed to the good life people appreciate today. San Jose Taiko member Wisa Uemura says the song is "really about gratitude . . . for what has had to happen to make what we have good and blessed."[44] "Ei Ja Nai Ka?" combines drumming, singing, *kakegoe* (chanting), and simple dance phrases that move in a circular pattern. Hirabayashi created the dance, drum, and kakegoe parts in 1994 and in 2001 asked Yoko Fujimoto, a folksinger, member of the Japanese performing arts troupe Hanayui, and former member of Kodo, to write a melody and lyrics to accompany the dance.[45] The work is performed widely as part of San Jose Taiko's touring repertoire, and it is also familiar to many taiko players because of the North American Taiko Conference, as indicated in the introduction to this chapter. San Jose Taiko teaches it to other taiko groups that want to learn and perform it for their own communities.

Whereas the musical and gestural vocabulary are inspired by contemporary Japanese folk performance, the piece is also a staple in the San Jose Obon repertoire of *bon* dances, which are part of obon, the Buddhist festival honoring the dead.[46] The content of the piece draws on an aspect of the Japanese American past, but its form is inspired by music and dance conventions that are currently practiced in Japan and in Japanese American communities, and in keeping with obon sensibilities, its tone is both somber and joyful as it brings the past and present together in performance.[47] In *bon-odori*, or festival dances, a drummer and flutist accompany dancers who move in repeated patterns, usually in a circle or in lines. Inspired by the Japanese folk arts group Warabi-za and by the traditions of Kyushu's Kokura Gion Matsuri and Awa Odori of Shikoku, Hirabayashi began to contemplate a folk dance piece that would be unique to San Jose Taiko and that would reflect a Japanese diasporic experience.[48] While it is fairly common for taiko groups to participate in obon or other festival dances by either giving a concert or playing the drum parts for the large group dances, "Ei Ja Nai Ka?" is unique in that it was created for San Jose Taiko to perform as well as to teach to taiko players and nonplayers, Asian American or not. It is highly participatory because, while the group members always perform the piece, festival-goers are encouraged to join in the dance circle (see figure 2.3).

As a participant in the dance, I embody in the present the labors of early Japanese immigrants. Although Japanese laborers supported themselves in a number of ways, including business and entrepreneurship, "Ei Ja Nai Ka?" focuses on manual labor, including gestures that mimic digging, picking (as if in a mine), fishing, steering, and wiping the sweat from one's brow. When San Jose Taiko members perform these movements, they have a crisp yet buoyant energy. As they dig and pick, they sing the call and response: "Ei Ja Nai Ka!" "A So-re, A So-re!" "Ei Ja Nai Ka, hai!" "A So-re, So-re, Yoi-sho!"[49] As I stumble through the movements, I have to remind myself of the choreography, repeating, "Dig, dig / Pick, pick," in my head as I step sharply with my right foot on the first and second beats ("Dig, dig"), while jutting my fisted hands down and to the right, as if I'm thrusting a shovel into the earth. On beats three and four ("Pick, pick") I step sharply to the left and raise my arms above head, jutting my imaginary pickax into the mine wall above my head. Song lyrics that accompany the drumming, chanting, and dancing refer to the physical

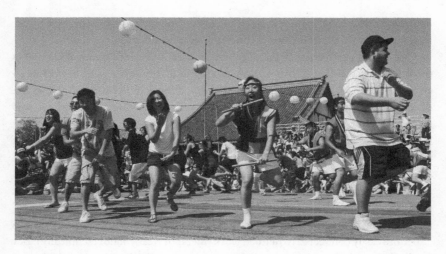

Figure 2.3. San Jose Taiko in performance at the San Jose Obon Festival. Yurika Chiba leads festival dancers in "Ei Ja Nai Ka?" www.taiko.org. Photo by Higashi Design. Used with permission.

effects—dyed fingers and "stretched" backs—of harvesting strawberries in the field. These gestures and lyrics point to the kinds of work the issei performed. Japanese immigration began in earnest in the 1880s, when Japanese workers, both men and women, came to the United States to labor on farms and railroads and in mills and mines. It was largely halted in 1907 after Emperor Mutsuhito and President Theodore Roosevelt created the Gentlemen's Agreement that effectively barred Japanese immigration. After the passing of the Alien Land Laws, issei farmers barred from owning land were forced to move every two or three years. Many continued the back-breaking "stoop" labor throughout their lives, while others created their own businesses. Between 1900 and 1909, Japanese-owned businesses boomed. Despite these successes the issei faced racial discrimination, as had Chinese and Filipino laborers before them. Few spoke English or had access to education, and efforts to establish anti-racist labor unions failed. By 1913, lawmakers sought to halt the opening of more Japanese-owned businesses and farms.[50]

Throughout the lyrics, which are sung in Japanese, the singer-narrator is figured as someone in the present time speaking to earlier generations. The song literally addresses "Grandpa" and "Grandma," though one might also take those monikers to be figurative of ancestors, rather than literal references to lineage: "Ei ja nai ka, ei ja nai ka, Grandpa, ei ja nai ka? / Ei ja nai ka, ei ja nai ka, Grandma, ei ja nai ka?"[51] "Grandpa" and "Grandma" are sung in Japanese pronunciation with four syllables: "Gu-ra-n-ma" and "Gu-ra-n-pa." This line solidifies the song's dedication to the issei using direct address and asking, essentially, wasn't the sacrifice—the "sweat dripping"—worthwhile? As Asian American historian Ron Takaki points out, issei came to be thought of as immigrants only in retrospect, since many came as temporary laborers, only to see their options for returning to Japan dwindle once they arrived on U.S. shores.[52] They may have dreamed of returning to their homeland rather than beginning a new life in the United States, but this lyric none-theless recognizes the hardships of their early years in the country.

One of the most expansive movement phrases, the steering move, highlights the way "Ei Ja Nai Ka?" elevates manual labor to an honored—and honorable—symbol of progress. Hirabayashi notes that one gesture in the song, in which the dancer spreads her arms wide and rotates them as if steering a giant wheel, was inspired by her grandfather's work as an engine wiper on the Southern Pacific Railroad: "Engine wiper sounds like a very menial and almost demeaning type of position, but . . . it's that kind of labor that has built this nation."[53] In a workshop she demonstrates the effects that this labor had on her grandfather by bending forward at the waist, explaining that her grandfather's back was permanently hunched. The shift from the position of engine wiper to steering is more than simply a wishful revision of history. On one level, steering is a more legible gesture than wiping and also more easily connected to railroad work (metaphorically, if not technically). But for the dancer, this steering motion requires more than the limited range of driving an imaginary car. In order to steer this train, I spread my arms full-length to each side, hands fisted, and tilt forty-five degrees with a bent right knee and straight left leg, the horizontal arms tilting along my body's line. I repeat this motion to the left, and once more on each side. The steering motion is the simplest and broadest of the dance, requiring me to extend my body to its limits. Each tilt is punctuated with a shouted phrase: "EI! JA! NAI! KA!" It is a full and celebratory movement, one that is pleasurable to execute. It transforms exploited physical laborers into powerful leaders performing rewarding work, and though it accomplishes this by a revision of history, the gesture (both the physical movement and the sentiment) highlights how crucial issei labor was to the industrial and economic progress of the nation.

The railroad imagery in the lyrics is explicitly tied to notions of progress:

> Smoke puffs out, making a roar
> A sora ei ja nai ka—Railroad—ei ja nai ka
> Ei ja nai ka—Steam engine—ei ja nai ka
> The railroad expands from west to east,
> Carrying today's load toward tomorrow.[54]

In accounts of Asian American history, the railroad is most commonly associated with Chinese American labor, specifically the vast numbers of Chinese laborers who built the Central Pacific Railroad, only to be erased from mainstream histories' commemorations of this remarkable achievement. But as many as ten thousand Japanese laborers worked on railroads in 1909, suffering under harsh labor conditions and extreme temperatures.[55] The railroad can be read as a symbol of achievement and national progress. Asian American histories generally mark railroad labor as a site of unfair labor practices. "Ei Ja Nai Ka?" honors the labor of issei railroad workers and uses the railroad as a symbol of a different kind of progress. Here, perhaps, the railroad symbolizes progress toward equality and justice for Japanese immigrants, rather than industrial achievement. On the other hand, viewing Japanese Americans' part in American industrial achievement may itself be a vehicle for racial progress.

"Ei Ja Nai Ka?" frames issei struggles as ones that were overcome and resulted in the success of future generations. Yet historian Yuji Ichioka has argued that the struggle for survival was "far from being a success story."[56] Japanese laborers, like those from Mexico and other parts of Asia, worked under harsh conditions, including extreme cold and hot temperatures, insufficient lodging, and long hours, among other injustices.[57] But the fervent racism that many issei suffered goes unmentioned in this song. Further, the focus on agricultural and industrial labor belies the fact that many issei became successful merchants who founded businesses small and large during the first decade of the 1900s. In 1910, there was roughly one business per twenty-two people within the Japanese population of the western United States.[58] Moreover, household duties fell on the shoulders of women in addition to their jobs, leaving them with a double workload.[59] While "Ei Ja Nai Ka?" highlights pre-internment manual labor, the song's celebration of racial and community progress eclipses other aspects of Japanese American history.

Hirabayashi and San Jose Taiko are well aware of that past and are very likely also aware of the pitfalls of ascribing it to a teleological history. The internment of 110,000 Japanese and Japanese Americans during World War II is clear evidence that racial progress is not linear. Many taiko groups have songs about or dedicated to this dark chapter of Japanese American history or reference the event as a kind of originary moment from which American taiko has proceeded. That this piece notably omits internment indicates that the piece has more to do with the connections between the issei and sansei than it does with relating a complete and accurate timeline of Japanese American history. As member Wisa Uemura says, the song recognizes "the first Issei coming to this country, [and] that we can benefit from even playing taiko is from their hard work."[60] The song acknowledges the issei for the economic and social foundations they provided for later generations' successes, achievements, and leisure.

In festival settings, where all of the elements repeat for an unspecified length of time and the purpose is to join in the dancing and chanting, the kinesthetic aspects of participating in the dance take precedence. At the North American Taiko Conference, taking part in the dancing, drumming, chanting, and singing that comprise this piece reminds taiko players—many of whom are not Japanese American or Asian American—that our ability to practice taiko at all is due to Asian American activism and the parents and grandparents whose labor made this elaborate leisure activity possible in the first place. In that context, "Ei Ja Nai Ka?" teaches Asian American history to taiko players with a range of backgrounds and investments in the form.[61] When San Jose Taiko performs at the San Jose obon festival, perhaps some of the effects are similar. In the context of a Japantown event, the work may speak more directly to Japanese Americans, Asian Americans, or those who have a specific connection to those communities. In both situations, the piece affords people the opportunity to move together in the present moment and engage with the past through the shared labors of dancing, singing, and chanting.

The significance of "Ei Ja Nai Ka?" in San Jose Taiko's repertoire is evidenced not only by its being widely taught but also by its inclusion in the group's thirty-fifth anniversary concert, recorded on DVD in 2009. In this abbreviated version of the piece, the progress narrative is made more obvious by cutting the middle verses of the lyrics dedicated to specific types of labor, and the audience participation elements are reduced because the piece is performed in a proscenium auditorium rather than in a festival setting. The anniversary arrangement begins at a slow and somber pace, emphasizing laborious movement, and proceeds to a fast, celebratory dance. These aspects seem appropriate to an anniversary concert celebrating the group's longevity, but I am interested in how this shortened version, as embodied history, emphasizes teleology and the notion of progress. Moving from slow to fast, mournful to celebratory, dark to light, this arrangement gestures to the memory of sacrifice and labor in order to celebrate the fruits of that labor in the present.

The piece begins with the stage bare except for two *chu-daiko* (medium-sized barrel drums) standing upright stage left and stage right in front of a red cyclorama. Slow single beats on the *atarigane*, a metal hand gong, precede one performer's entrance. The atarigane player begins to sing as the performer slowly enters from stage left and stands still on the platform that stretches across the upstage area. Almost as soon as she initiates the song, the voices of the company join hers from offstage. Four men enter from stage right, four heavy left feet landing in time with the atarigane's slow beats. They continue to put one foot in front of the other. They grasp their bachi with both hands, as if holding the handle of an axe, and as they begin each step, their arms hoist the bachi above their heads, and then let the imaginary weight of the axe pull their arms down. They are working on a railroad, in a chain gang. One of the men pushes a drum onstage as though it is filled with lead. They continue across the stage, and once in place stage left, they root their feet in a wide stance and continue, now in canon round, to swing their axes. Meanwhile, three performers enter stage left, singing, facing the audience, stepping sideways as they plant rice with their hands. Holding *uchiwa* (hand-held fan drums) in their left hands, they use their right hands to dip into their uchiwa as if they are baskets. In time to the music they pick seeds and throw them, pick and throw, then pick and bend down to plant them, and finally pick and scatter the seeds. Their eyes, like the railroad workers', are downcast, concentrating on their labor.

After several beats the long introduction ends, and the energy shifts subtly. All the dancers continue their gestures but now have a slight bounce in their feet, as if some new energy has sprung up through the ground into their bodies. Two or three people shout kakegoe: "Hai!" "Za!" Soon the somber formality dissolves, and the performers scatter into different positions: the railroad workers wipe the sweat from their brows, roll drums downstage, and begin to play. The rice planters beat their uchiwa as they leap and chant. Wisa Uemura and P. J. Hirabayashi enter upstage right with a large *okedo* drum on wheels, which they begin to beat with buoyant energy. Drummer Franco Imperial sets a *shime-daiko* down upstage left and smiles as he lays down a peppy swing beat. The chu-daiko players perform one round of the drum melody, then the uchiwa players rush downstage, each taking brief solos down center. This section has the informal feel of an impromptu jam session. It is a familiar taiko composition format: play the "song" and then allow for short virtuosic solos. But in the context of the song's focus on labor, it also is reminiscent of laborers' impromptu entertainments, showing off for each other with their individual moves as an appreciative crowd looks on.

The company crescendos through a long chant of "So-re, so-re, so-re, so-re, so-re, so-re, so-re, so-re!" and scatters once again into another formation. Imperial, Hirabayashi, and Uemura continue to drum on the upstage platform and are now joined by three uchiwa players. All the other performers form a circle on the main stage and begin the folk dance as they sing the melody again: Dig and pick, roll and sweat, steer, steer. This setup mirrors as closely as it can the festival version of the song: the musicians accompany the dancers, and they all sing together. They run through the dance twice and then re-form into two lines facing the audience. They dance, some sing, and some chant. Here, all parts of "Ei Ja Nai Ka?" come together in all its complexity. By this point in the performance, although the labor is still present in the dance gestures, it is layered with so many songs, chants, and beats that it is woven into a celebratory cacophony. The lighting is brighter, the pace is faster, and the dancers move with the signature San Jose Taiko bounce, glittering smiles on all their faces. The piece ends abruptly as the melody, dance, and chant end. As the last line of the lyrics, "Tatako yo, Odoro yo!" ("Let's beat the taiko! Let's dance!") is sung, the dancers hoist imaginary fishing nets toward the audience, pointing their bachi right at them, and shout a final "Yoi-sho!"

This version of the piece omits the lyrics that focus on the types of issei labor and skips to an ending verse that celebrates dancing and drumming. But even if spectators could not recognize the Japanese lyrics, the brevity of the piece, along with its dramatic shifts, suggests a celebratory teleology. "Ei Ja Nai Ka?" as staged in this DVD performance conveys a triumphant success for Japanese Americans and for the United States. The piece draws on Japanese performance traditions, world music influences, and the diasporic tradition of the obon festival to re-member and revise our understanding of Japanese immigration and intergenerational dynamics. This background may be familiar to San Jose Taiko's Asian American audiences, but this story of racial progress may be new to mainstream audiences in the United States and abroad. As the piece continues to be performed today, its celebration of immigrant labor resonates against a cacophony of politicians voicing hostility, fear, and violent rhetoric toward immigrants in the United States. By late 2017 it was clear that rhetoric has shifted to physical and legislative violence toward immigrants such as the white supremacist march in Charlottesville, Virginia, President Donald Trump's announcement of his intention to end the Obama-era Dreamers Act, and his repeated attempts to enact an immigration ban on seven countries with majority Muslim populations, which the long-standing Japanese American Citizens League continues to oppose.[62]

The creation of Japanese American histories, whether through writing or performance, not only connects issei to sansei, past to present, but also connects San Jose Taiko to the Asian American movement itself. The writing of such histories has been instrumental in AAM politics, given the movement's involvement in the creation of ethnic studies programs in California colleges. Josephine Lee connects these impulses to those that have shaped plays that evoke Asian American histories as well: "The eagerness to write history points to the desire for an authenticating past that will support a communal future; within the enactment of the meticulous details of history are purposes that shape theatrical presentation."[63]"Ei Ja Nai Ka?" enacts a revision of the past via gesture and sound in ways that not only complement and extend written histories of Asian America but that also encourage a "communal future" in which all willingly participate in and remember those histories as a route to structural equality and social justice.

MARKETING ASIAN AMERICAN TAIKO: BETWEEN WORLD DANCE AND ACTIVISM

When San Jose Taiko performed at the Long Center for the Performing Arts in Austin, Texas, on September 27, 2009, the last number did not end in the usual way, with bows and quick exits. Rather, it only ended after the entire ensemble danced down the aisles through the applauding audience, still playing instruments—small hand-held gongs, cymbals, and large drums strapped to their bodies—smiling and shouting spirited cries along with the rhythms. Once they arrived in the large, glass-fronted lobby that overlooks the river and the colorfully lit buildings of downtown Austin, the players positioned themselves strategically throughout the space so that they could greet as many departing audience members as possible. Rather than disappearing backstage and exiting in street clothes much later, San Jose Taiko members routinely talk with audiences while the labor of their performance is still evident: they appear with rumpled costumes and sweaty skin, their breathing still heavy from performing. They are approachable and warm as they shake many hands, accept congratulations, and answer questions for almost an hour after the performance has ended.[64] Bringing the performance out into the house and greeting their audiences in the lobby, even in the formal setting of a large performing venue, is part of how San Jose Taiko reaches out to communities when they tour nationally and internationally.

Gathered around P. J. Hirabayashi in a cluster by the large windows was a group of local taiko players. They were identifiable as such because they sported sweatshirts and t-shirts with the names of their groups, Austin Taiko and Kaminari Taiko (of Houston) and because they were chatting with Hirabayashi about workshops that have been scheduled in Austin later that week. In another spot near the theater doors, Franco Imperial spoke animatedly with interested audience members, some of whom, I later learned, are relatives of his who live in the Austin area. Around the lobby, several other group members fielded questions and compliments from a range of people: tall white Texan men in dress jeans and cowboy boots, young women in high heels, and couples leading their children by the hand. Other San Jose Taiko members obligingly signed the programs of the many Asian and Latino/a children standing in line for their autographs. The crowd that San Jose Taiko has drawn was decidedly more racially diverse than audiences at other Long Center performances such as the ballet, the symphony, and other national touring shows, and the presenter's brochures have been designed to attract crowds interested in performances that lie outside the European and American canon.

Despite San Jose Taiko's complex understanding of its grounding in Asian American politics and history, presenters often rely on Orientalist rhetoric to promote the group's shows. In some cases its performances are imagined as Japanese, rather than Asian American. Much of the group's work for four decades has been to make Asian Americans legible—visually and sonically—in a variety of contexts. Taiko players in the 1960s and 1970s often saw taiko as a way to replace negative images of stereotyped Orientals with a more active and positive picture of themselves. In part, San Jose Taiko's adopting an Asian American stance was a way to distinguish the group from Japanese taiko groups, as well as to acknowledge the different histories and experiences of Japanese and Asian American people. Current members are clearly still invested in these aims. In some performance contexts, San Jose Taiko can articulate its history, influences, and philosophical aims. At some large performance venues, some of this ability falls under the control of presenters' marketing departments and PR materials.

The brochure announcing the 2009–2010 season of the Long Center for the Performing Arts sports a montage of its varied offerings: classical music, dance, musical theater, and more.[65] The Long Center, which opened in 2008, is home to Austin's ballet company, symphony orchestra, and opera company and presents a variety of national touring performances. In 2009 San Jose Taiko was among them, and a slice of the cover montage was accordingly filled with a San Jose Taiko image. Wisa Uemura is dressed in a happi coat and hachimaki, her face and left arm reaching skyward against a deep red background. Uemura's smiling face is lit brightly, and the rim of a chu-daiko almost fades into the adjacent photograph. To the left of Uemura is a black-and-white photo of classical pianist Lang Lang gazing philosophically skyward, and to the right, the actors playing Danny and Sandy in the musical Grease grin happily from the cover. Inside the brochure, San Jose Taiko's performances are listed as part of the "International" series.

San Jose Taiko's positioning in these marketing materials exemplifies what dance studies scholar Susan Foster calls the "worlding" of dance. Foster argues that although the term "world" as applied to music, dance, and other arts purports to view all performance as equal under one category ("the world"), the "colonial history that produced [the imbalance] continues to operate" in practice. Reading a brochure for the 2007–2008 Cal Performances at the University of California, Berkeley, Foster notes that only ballet and modern companies, consisting mainly of white people, qualify as "Dance," whereas performance by artists of color are "World Dance."[66] In a similar fashion, the Long Center's season brochure relegates its performances by artists of color to the two categories "Dance with a Difference" and "International." The other categories—"Broadway," "Off-Broadway," "Classical Variations," "Musical Legends," and "Specials"—present work created and performed by white artists, with the exception of Lang Lang, the Chinese pianist whose repertoire of European classical music qualifies him as simply an artist. The "Dance with a Difference" category includes the presumably Latin-influenced, "sizzling" Ballroom with a Twist and the hiphop show Groovaloo, while the "International" category includes San Jose Taiko, the Ballet Folklorico de Mexico and Spirit of Uganda. San Jose Taiko is clearly not an international group when presented in the United States, but its inclusion among performances from Mexico and Uganda that blend dance and music is not surprising. Recordings of taiko music are often shelved as world music, and San Jose Taiko does, indeed, draw on musical traditions from around the world, including Latin and African music.

Nonetheless, the placement of San Jose Taiko in the International series disregards the long history of taiko as an American performance tradition and reinforces the designation of Asian Americans as perpetual foreigners. When the group tours nationally, presenters and agents capitalize on the ongoing commercial appeal of Asia as a cultural product by selling San Jose Taiko as "authentically" Japanese from "over there," rather than Asian American from San Jose, California. The image and copy that accompany San Jose's advertisement within the season brochure create what Emily Roxworthy calls a "theatricalizing discourse" about the group. Theatricalizing discourse presumes the maskedness and aesthetic distantness of Japanese people.[67] The brochure copy reads:

> These empowering and overwhelming sounds weave traditional Japanese music with the beat of world rhythms. It's extreme physical endurance, amazing theatrics and an [sic] transformative spirit that inspired an Empire. This is Taiko, a culture unseen for centuries and filled with the rituals of 5000 years. Percussionists will battle.[68]

Even if we dispense with the factual and grammatical errors in this blurb (modern taiko does not date back five thousand years, nor is it a competitive or "battle" performance style), the text characterizes taiko as something ancient ("unseen for centuries") and ritualized. The notions that taiko inspired an empire and that percussionists will battle are pure fantasy. That this particular group, which clearly and consistently emphasizes its connection to Japanese American communities and Asian American movement politics rooted in peace and equality, should be cast in such a mystical and militant light is indicative of the theatricalizing impulse of American culture.

The image against which the blurb is set reinforces the text's positioning of taiko as an ancient and exotic art form. Three drummers are shown in shadow against a luminous blue cyclorama—black, faceless figures with their arms held at forty-five-degree angles, about to strike the drums. The figures loom large against the backdrop, their shoulders broadened by the cut of the happi coats, any personal expression or detail obscured by the lighting technology. The performers' slender arms and silhouettes make them discernible as female, and the overall image, in concert with the text, makes the performers appear ominous, almost warriorlike. Although the Long Center appears to have edited the image only slightly, browsing San Jose Taiko's press and publicity Web page reveals that the Long Center likely chose the only image out of thirty-three that obscures, rather than highlights, performers' facial expressions and colorful costumes.

When I asked San Jose Taiko members about marketing materials in our interview, they laughed knowingly. About this particular brochure, Wisa Uemura said that whereas the copy emphasized the ancient and traditional, "we tend to not think of ourselves as traditional. We are definitely a contemporary taiko company . . . [the blurb is] not from any of our wording." Franco Imperial acknowledged that when the group's staff pointed out the problems with it, the Long Center had graciously changed the offending copy online but were unable to change the printed brochure because of deadlines.[69] The group does provide presenters' PR and marketing departments with Web access to extensive group histories, descriptions, program lineups, images, and video, but whether this information is passed along to the appropriate staff member is often out of San Jose Taiko's control. Perhaps part of the conundrum is that the Long Center's impulse to frame taiko as part of an unbroken lineage dating back thousands of years taps into their audience's wish for authenticity. That many players, Asian American or not, see taiko in Japan as authoritative and seek training and inspiration from their Japanese counterparts complicates this issue.

The Orientalist leanings of advertising and marketing are not new to San Jose Taiko. Roy and P. J. Hirabayashi both stated that in the past, agents and presenters have urged them to change the group's name, either to something "sexier" or to "something Japanese." Roy also noted that, particularly in areas with relatively few Asian Americans, "they're trying to represent us as a group from Japan. . . . And then the audience kind of thinks that's what we are when we really feel that we're trying to present a more American or Asian American perspective to what taiko's all about." As San Jose Taiko tries to differentiate itself from taiko groups from Japan who are, essentially, its competition, the very avenues through which to do so (agents and marketing departments) urge it to become *more like* other taiko groups, once again collapsing the difference between Asian and Asian American.

San Jose Taiko does not compromise its aesthetic or ideals by bending to Orientalist demands; it attempts to distinguish itself from other touring taiko groups. Franco Imperial said that in contrast to Kodo, which maintains a kind of "mystique" within and around its performances, San Jose Taiko makes an effort to connect with its audience. Group members carry their performance offstage, dissolving the distance between audience and performer. Imperial stated that this is all part of San Jose Taiko's "emotional accessibility."

Outside the touring venue, the group tries "as much as possible to connect with the local [taiko] groups." Although San Jose Taiko's full-scale concerts usually take place in cities with large venues, it also performs school shows in more rural or remote areas, many of whose populations include very few Asian Americans or other racial minorities. Wisa Uemura mentioned that in schools, particularly where there may be very little exposure to Asian people or cultures, group members may seem "different," but they "make 'different' cool . . . accessible, and acceptable." Meg Suzuki added that when audiences include very few Asian Americans, she feels particularly motivated to reach out to them:

> I wish I could say, you know, like, "I actually grew up in rural Pennsylvania. . . . I'm like you!" I didn't know what other Asians, gosh, looked like even. It was just me. I mean, I lived in a place where the Klan came through town every once in a while, you know? Like, I wish there was some point where I could be like, "I know what you're feeling. I feel your pain. It's going to be okay."

Both Uemura and Suzuki, like other members of San Jose Taiko, are invested in using taiko to connect with the communities in which they perform. In some instances, this means teaching their audiences to respect racial difference, while in others, it means reaching out to Asians and Asian Americans who might feel isolated in rural or largely white areas, a topic I explore in more depth in Chapter 3.

Performances and encounters with audience members may in some instances disrupt the Orientalist rhetoric that pervades marketing materials and, too often, audiences' perspectives, but they continue to be sites of negotiation and even struggle for San Jose Taiko and other groups. These sometimes seemingly futile attempts to redirect spectators' Orientalist impulses via audience engagement are part of the complex constellation of identities and influences that San Jose Taiko navigates as an Asian American, Japanese American, and multiethnic performance ensemble in the United States.

Group members continue to shape and be shaped by Asian American movement politics through their enactment of embodied Asian American histories, organizational structure, and continued struggles with Orientalist representation. In negotiating Japanese authenticity, Asian American activism, and multiple artistic influences, San Jose Taiko has also deeply influenced the trajectory of North American taiko. The organizational structure of the group reflects the founders' involvement with the Asian American movement. Moreover, the group's leadership within the taiko community and P. J. and Roy's extensive leadership outside the group makes it clear that San Jose Taiko's influence has extended well beyond the heyday of political activism in the 1970s. Because it has been so widely taught and performed, "Ei Ja Nai Ka?" and its ability to connect audiences and participants with Asian American history has also carried out AAM ideals through performance. Finally, the group's negotiation of exoticizing and Orientalist assumptions on the part of presenters and marketing departments highlights the continuing necessity of carrying out messages that early Asian American movement activists and pioneer taiko players brought to light. Not all taiko groups give as much explicit attention to the structural, political, and representational aspects of taiko as does San Jose Taiko, but all North American taiko players must move through this tangle of performance, politics, and everyday life. The performers featured in Chapter 3 navigate the racial terrain of Minnesota, whose Asian American communities and racial landscape differ from many areas of California. This chapter turns to the Midwest in its exploration of Minneapolis-based Mu Daiko and more explicitly to outreach performance, an area of performance studies that, though undertheorized, forms an important part of many performing arts groups. Outreach—giving small-scale performances in corporate and educational venues to develop an audience and deepen educational experiences—constitutes a large portion of Mu Daiko's activities and elucidate issues of race and racial knowledge.

CHAPTER 3

Taiko Scenarios

Performing Asian America in the Land of 10,000 Lakes

When I moved from Minnesota to Texas in 2006, I had been performing and teaching taiko classes with the Minneapolis-based taiko group Mu Daiko for several years, and one of my students gave me a Minnesota snow globe as a going-away present. Encased in the glass orb are Paul Bunyan and Babe the Blue Ox, the giant lumberjack and his bovine companion who, according to folklore, created the state's 10,000 lakes with their footprints. They are joined by the state bird, the black-and-white feathered loon, and the eponymous Minnesota lake cabin nestled amid tall pine trees. And of course, there's the snow. I could almost step into the globe myself, since white, blond, blue-eyed Scandinavians are as much a part of the state's imaginary as the loon and the lakes. Despite its increasingly diverse population, the state of Minnesota maintains an investment in its whiteness, in part through long-running cultural productions like *A Prairie Home Companion*, in which the "true" Minnesota lies in the fictional Lake Wobegon's Lutheran church potlucks and Scandinavian-inflected long Os.[1] In reality, however, the state is by no means uniformly white. Particularly in the twin cities of Minneapolis and St. Paul, the racial landscape is heterogeneous, with significant populations of Somali Americans, Latino/as, and American Indians. Minnesota is also home to the nation's largest concentration of adopted Koreans and the second-largest concentration of Hmong Americans, and during the 1980s and 1990s the state's overall Asian population roughly doubled.[2]

In this chapter I use taiko outreach performance to better understand Asian American racial formations in Minnesota. Through ethnographic participant-observation, autoethnographic reflection, and performance analysis I highlight the textural, sensory, lived experiences of those performing Asian America in an apparently culturally white region. Considering Minnesota's racial landscape through the lens of Asian Americanist performance interrupts the black-white framing of racism nationally and in the Midwest, and the demographic make-up of Mu Daiko highlights one of the state's most statistically significant yet figuratively invisible, populations, adopted Korean Americans. Mu Daiko emerged as part of Theater Mu, an Asian American performing arts group that has grown considerably and exerted a major influence on the theatrical landscape of Minneapolis–St. Paul since its founding in 1992. Part of the success of the company, renamed Mu Performing Arts in 2001, has been what the company considers "outreach performance," low-tech engagements with an educational focus, often with a goal of introducing audiences to Asian and Asian American performance. Although the distinction between fully produced taiko concerts and taiko outreach performance is somewhat arbitrary, it is how Mu Daiko members distinguished the kinds of educational engagements that required only a few performers from the more formal and higher-stakes annual concerts that showcased the full membership. Focusing on outreach is important because the practice brings performers into contact with audiences who might not typically attend more expensive concerts in Minneapolis or St. Paul, and it thus encourages interactions between performers and a broader range of audiences.

A rich site for examining everyday embodied knowledge about race, Mu Daiko outreach performance complicates familiar ideas about "Minnesota," imagined largely as white, and about "Asian America," often figured as a series of tightly knit enclaves on the West and East Coasts of the United States. On Minnesota's stages, as well as on the edges of cafeterias, in conference rooms, and in gymnasiums, Mu Daiko's outreach demonstrates the ways Asian Americans are seen, in Karen Shimakawa's terms, as "abject": constituting part of the nation and also demonstrating the limits of a coherent, unified whole. According to this view, Asian Americans are present in, but not always seen as part of, American culture.[3] Minneapolis–St. Paul (the Twin Cities, to locals), a major metropolitan area in the Midwest, is not monolithically white, yet its Asian American communities differ from those on the West Coast. Nonetheless, taiko outreach brings Mu Daiko members into contact with urban and rural communities throughout the Midwest, and their experiences complicate received understandings of the region.[4] As I demonstrate, Mu Daiko's racially mixed membership and outreach experiences show that the Midwest and its Asian American communities are complex entities and that the cultural production at the crossroads of Minnesota and Asian America deserves greater critical attention.

Viewing racial formation in Minnesota through the lens of performance requires thinking about the gestural and embodied dimensions of race. In her powerful anthology *A Good Time for the Truth: Race in Minnesota,* editor Sun Yung Shin asks, "People of color are the fastest growing segment of Minnesota's population. But is Minnesota a state that understands 'race'?"[5] In this chapter I consider not simply *whether* the state understands race, but also *how* Minnesotans (including Mu Daiko members) understand and perform their racial knowledge. Mu Daiko's seemingly simple outreach performances enable complex avenues of spectatorship, identification, and cross-racial encounter within a Midwestern context. Because outreach performances require a degree of improvisation—that is, they are based on a loosely scripted scenario that performers modify for particular circumstances—they open up possibilities for returning the audience's gaze and performing Asian America in new ways on and off stage. Audiences, too, bring their own embodied knowledge to the performance scenario, and by attending to audience interactions, I demonstrate how Mu Daiko members negotiate and respond to encounters that range from the obviously racist to transformative connections.

In what follows, I first provide a brief history and overview of Mu Daiko, its members, and the function of outreach performance. I then deepen the discussion of outreach by deploying Diana Taylor's notions of "repertoire" and "scenario" as critical lenses through which to understand how performance—on the stage and in everyday life—transmits cultural knowledge, often without the performers' or audience's awareness. With this critical lens in place, I proceed to three readings. In the first, through interview analysis, I examine how Mu Daiko negotiates issues of race, identity, and emotional labor on the organizational and individual levels. Next, using part of my interview with Mu Daiko member Susie Kuniyoshi, I think through the ways Minnesotans and others rely on what Robin Bernstein calls "racial innocence" to deflect charges of racism. I ask how innocence, "a performance of not-noticing," works alongside a repertoire of racist gestures to uphold the status quo.[6] Finally, I turn to the interviews and spoken-word performance of group members who are Korean American adoptees to consider how Mu Daiko outreach enables connection between these performers and audience members, unsettling the very Orientalist frameworks in which taiko is often presented. I argue that Mu Daiko outreach complicates easy definitions of Asian America and Minnesota and reveals both the pervasive racial attitudes of audience members and the repertoire of survival strategies that members use to negotiate such encounters.

MINNESOTA'S ASIAN AMERICA: MU DAIKO AND ITS MEMBERS

For twenty years, Mu Daiko has occupied the unique position of being a taiko group conjoined with an Asian American theater company in the Twin Cities. Although Mu Daiko was not the first taiko group in the state, it emerged as part of Minnesota's first Asian American theater company. In 2017 the theater and taiko sides of Mu Performing Arts split to pursue separate goals.[7] The seeds of Mu Daiko were sown when Rick Shiomi, at that time the artistic director of the fledgling Theater Mu, performed solo on a taiko drum for a fundraising event in 1997. Shiomi admits that when he, Martha Johnson, and Dong il-Lee founded Theater Mu in 1992 Minnesota had seemed to him an unlikely place in which to establish such a company. Having been involved in Asian American and Canadian theater, taiko, and community activism on the West Coast, he doubted that Minnesota's relatively small Asian American community could support a theater company. In what is by now a well-known anecdote, Shiomi describes walking up to Asians on the street and asking them if they wanted to be in a play, since he didn't know of any other way to find Asian American actors in Minnesota. Other Asian American arts and community groups existed in the Twin Cities at that time, but Mu became the first such theater company in Minnesota. It remains a successful company and celebrated its twenty-fifth anniversary in 2017.

When Mu Daiko was formed in 1997, taiko had already been established as a local practice more than a decade earlier. Kogen Taiko, a group connected to the Japanese American Buddhist taiko tradition, had begun performing in the Twin Cities in 1985.[8] Its membership was, for many years, restricted to people with family connections to its original members, however, and the group did not offer regular taiko classes.[9] In recent years, several new groups have formed in the area, most of them started by former Mu Daiko or Kogen players.[10]

Shiomi often says he never meant to start a taiko group in Minneapolis and that it was only at the insistence of a few regular Theater Mu actors that the group got off the ground.[11] Shiomi, who is Japanese Canadian, had been part of the wave of Canadian taiko groups to emerge in the late 1970s, inspired by the California-based groups San Jose Taiko, San Francisco Taiko Dojo, and Kinnara Taiko, as well as by the Japanese touring group Ondekoza, whose 1979 tour to North America inspired many Asian Americans and Asian Canadians with their virtuosic performances. He played taiko with several groups in the late 1970s and 1980s, including San Francisco Taiko Dojo, but his involvement in taiko tapered off when his playwriting career took off after the success of his first play, *Yellow Fever* (1982). When he assumed leadership of Theater Mu in 1993, he concentrated his energies on playwriting and running the company and did not actively pursue taiko.[12]

But when Theater Mu secured a new office and rehearsal space in 1997, Shiomi performed "Matsuri" ("Festival") at the housewarming party, and several Theater Mu actors were captivated by his performance. He had bought some taiko, thinking that they would come in handy sometime for the theater company. Although I was not there to witness it, I can imagine Rick performing in his serene and graceful style, arms arcing out around him between beats, bachi tapping the drum's wooden rims in the light *kara ka ka* refrain of "Matsuri." Jennifer Weir—a Mu actor who would become a taiko player—recalls, "It was one drum, one person, one simple song, and I just thought it was beautiful and engaging."[13] After the party, Weir and several others begged him to start teaching taiko.[14] With reluctance, Shiomi agreed, thinking, "Oh, this'll discourage them." But rather than finding taiko too challenging, they wanted to continue, and later that year, the group performed its first short concert.[15] At that time the group was comprised solely of Asian American players, mostly the actors who had convinced him to teach them. Whereas Rick had imagined that they would play one concert and taiko would recede from people's minds, his wife and Mu co-founder Martha Johnson convinced him that the group had potential. From that first concert, Mu Daiko grew quickly, offering classes and annual concerts.[16] By 2001 Theater Mu was restructured and renamed "Mu

Performing Arts" to reflect the contributions of Mu Daiko to the company's programming and financial stability.

The addition of the taiko group came at a time when Theater Mu was crafting an aesthetic that featured a "blending of Eastern and Western performance styles." As Hsiu-Chen Classon and Esther Kim Lee both note, in the late 1990s the company worked with a number of local Asian immigrant artists whose traditional Asian arts practices could be incorporated into Mu's shows.[17] Other Asian American theaters in the 1990s avoided using traditional Asian forms in their productions because they felt that doing so was self-Orientalizing, but Shiomi insists that "cutting yourself off from those cultural roots and those cultural forms" is a form of self-denial.[18] Taiko, as an Asian and Asian American folk art (albeit with twentieth-century roots), fit with the aesthetic of using so-called traditional Asian forms as a way of performing Asian America.

Mu Daiko's members come to taiko with a range of identities, ages, experiences, and reasons for playing taiko. The original group, pictured in figure 3.1, included members of Japanese, Korean, Indian, and Filipino descent. As the group began to recruit new members in about 1999 from classes that were open to the public, the racial makeup of the group began to shift, slowly incorporating white performers. (Figure 3.2 shows the group in 2001, at which point the membership was roughly half Asian American and half white.) The absence of non-Asian people of color in Mu Daiko is not particularly unusual for North American taiko groups, in which African Americans, Latina/os, and others participate at much lower rates than do white and Asian American players.[19] Women have consistently comprised half or more of the group's members, and queer-identified members have also been part of the group throughout its history. Mu Daiko has had members as young as sixteen, as well as those in their sixties. It is not surprising, given the group's origins, that many early members came to Mu Daiko as theater artists, including Su-Yoon Ko and me (Ko as an actor, and me as a stage manager), as well as original members Shiomi, Jennifer Weir, Zaraawar Mistry, Lia Rivamonte, and Sara Dejoras. Some came to the group as experienced musicians, others with backgrounds in martial arts or an interest in Japanese culture, as well as professional lives as educators, attorneys, and graphic designers, among other professions.[20]

People's motivations to participate in Mu Daiko vary as well; some involve connections with Japan, notions of home, and ways of exploring identity. Rachel Gorton (pictured in figure 3.2), for example, a white woman from Minnesota who taught English in Japan for three years before moving back to the Twin Cities, started playing taiko as a way to maintain a connection to her time in Japan. And, as I elaborate in Chapter 4, she also found taiko empowering as a woman and as "something different" that enlivened her image of herself as a white suburbanite.[21] Al Zdrazil, a former Mu Daiko member and a retired prosecutor, began playing taiko in the fall of 1998 after seeing Mu Daiko perform at a park in St. Paul. A white man born in Minnesota, his interest in taiko stemmed from the "power and the

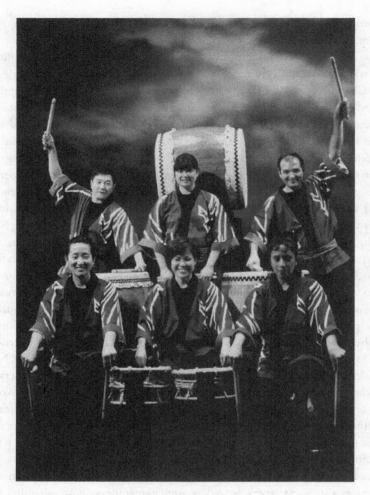

Figure 3.1. Mu Daiko poses for its second annual concert, "Thunder Drums of Mu Daiko," in December 1998. Front, left to right: Jennifer Weir, Iris Shiraishi, and Lia Rivamonte. Back, left to right: Rick Shiomi, Sara Dejoras, and Zaraawar Mistry. Photo by Charissa Uemura. Used with permission.

dynamism of it," as well as an interest in rhythm more generally. "For a long time," he said, he had been "fascinated by Japan." He in part developed this interest along with his daughter, who spent time going to Japanese language camp and traveling to Japan as a teenager.[22]

For some, therefore, taiko satisfies a desire for a Japanese culture that is far from home. For Asian American players it is a way to be "at home" in company with other Asian Americans. Susie Kuniyoshi was first welcomed into the group as a *fue* (Japanese flute) player while she held a post as a piccolo player with the Minnesota Orchestra; she later became the outreach director for Theater Mu. Born in Hilo, Hawai'i, she lived for many years on the East Coast and later in Duluth, Minnesota. Kuniyoshi said that her involvement with taiko, in particular her traveling to the

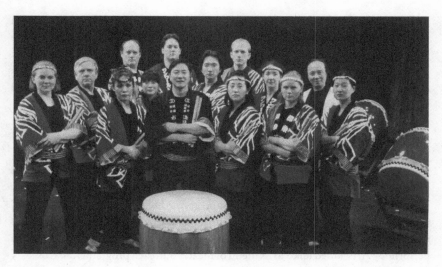

Figure 3.2. Mu Daiko poses for its fifth annual concert, "Spirit Drums: A Mu Daiko Concert," in December 2001. Left to right: Angela Ahlgren, Al Zdrazil, Iris Shiraishi, Patrick McCabe, Susie Kuniyoshi, Gregg Amundson, Rick Shiomi, Kiseung Rhee, Jennifer Weir, Drew Gorton (back), Laura Rawson, Rachel Gorton, Ying Zhang (guest flute artist), Su-Yoon Ko. Photo by Charissa Uemura. Used with permission.

North American Taiko Conference in 1999, made her feel more at home than she had felt in many years:

> I just remember the first taiko conference was an incredibly moving experience for me.... I felt like I came home ... maybe because I had been away for so long, and I had been living in northern Minnesota, where I felt completely displaced, you know. All of a sudden, I was sitting in this huge hall with all these people who were like me, who were Japanese American, um, from Hawai'i, not from Hawai'i, you know. So it was like this huge emotional thing.[23]

More than any other Mu Daiko member I interviewed, Susie articulates the ways in which taiko, especially large taiko gatherings where the majority of participants are Asian American, enables her to feel connected to Japanese American and Asian American communities. The feeling of "coming home," particularly for someone raised in largely Japanese American Hawai'i, was powerful enough that in recounting it to me a decade after the fact, she wiped tears from her eyes.

For other members, taiko's connection to Japanese culture is less of an end than a means to explore other aspects of Asian American identity. Su-Yoon Ko, a Korean American adoptee, played with Mu Daiko for several years before moving to South Korea, where she lived for eleven years. Ko said, "Studying taiko ... help[ed] spur me on to move to Korea to learn more about my own personal history. At some point I realized I knew more about Japan and Japanese culture than I did about Korea. And while I was happy to be learning about an Asian art form ... eventually

I felt ready to explore my own history and culture."[24] Ko added that, along with taiko, she had studied Kabuki, a classical Japanese theatrical form. While she enjoyed exploring art forms with roots in Japan for their own sake, they also forged a pathway for her to pursue her connection to her birth nation. Several of Mu Daiko's members are adopted Koreans who were raised in white Midwestern families, and I explore their experiences in more depth later in the chapter.

Taiko outreach allowed Mu Performing Arts to be competitive in Minneapolis's market for educational theater and has bolstered the company's operating budget. Though the outreach is designed to extend the company's mission to create "theater and taiko from the heart of the Asian American experience," it also benefits the company financially by bringing in revenue and increasing audience numbers.[25] Between 1997 and 2007 taiko alone constituted between 65 percent and 90 percent of all of Mu's outreach performances and averaged a total audience of between thirty-five thousand and forty-five thousand people annually.[26] Once Mu Performing Arts added taiko to its menu of theater outreach programs, taiko quickly became "an essential part of the growth engine of Mu."[27] As Shiomi explained, the programs, which included storytelling and short plays based on Asian American experiences, faced a lot of competition in the Minneapolis–St. Paul market. Because clients had so many educational theater programs to choose from, Mu's shows were only selected if the client had a specific desire to showcase Asian American material. But Mu Daiko created its own niche, one that no theater group could fill, and because Kogen Taiko only performed when its entire ensemble was available and Mu Daiko could send performers in small groups, the latter was, as Shiomi told me, essentially "the only game in town."[28] Mu's taiko outreach meets a need for Asian American educational performance, but it also has a potentially wider appeal than do the theater programs, focused as they are on specific identity-related issues. In other words, while taiko's history may be tied to Asian American identity and politics, it can also be read as simply Japanese or pan-Asian performance without the perceived cultural baggage of race and identity politics that may come with the self-narration of theater performance. Of course, as I explore in the next section, the slippage between Asian American, Japanese, and pan-Asian identities that broadens taiko's appeal also makes Mu Daiko outreach performers susceptible to Orientalist interpretations.

These engagements are flexible enough to operate in an arts ecology with a variety of demands related to race, ethnicity, and multiculturalism. As historian Vijay Prashad writes, multiculturalism is often "practiced [in the United States] as the *management* of diversity" (my italics), undercutting anti-racist sentiment. Thus, he states, "the history of oppression and the fact of exploitation are shunted aside in favor of a celebration of difference and the experience of individuals who can narrate their ethnicity for the consumption of others."[29] According to Susie Kuniyoshi, who served as the outreach director from 1999 to 2011, most clients offer one of three reasons for booking Mu; the client's enthusiasm for taiko as an art form is only the third most common. The two most common reasons are that clients "have a predominantly white demographic and they want to introduce their audience to a culture outside of their own . . . or . . . they have an Asian population and they want us to provide role models and self-validation to the audience."[30] These two seemingly contradictory goals—cultural enrichment for white audiences and providing role models for Asian American students—both deploy taiko as a corrective to a lack of racial diversity. Most of Mu Daiko's taiko outreach, then, is always already operating within a frame of multiculturalism, as a supplement or correction to pervasive whiteness, either that of the audience or of Minnesota more generally. Sometimes a client's impulse to provide a culture that is not the audience's own creates a scenario in which the audience is imagined (if not wholly constituted) as white and the performers are presented as exotic others. At other times the group is there to provide role models for Asian Americans in the audience who attend a school or live in a city, state, and ultimately a nation that is driven by a white majority, and taiko gives them access to a powerful performance form, presumably (but not always) performed by other Asian Americans.

Although group members come to taiko for a variety of reasons and from a range of backgrounds, performance contexts can sometimes flatten these complexities. At other times, however, performance sites open up space for the negotiation of identities. Looking closely at performances as well as off-stage encounters between performers and audiences reveals pervasive attitudes about Asians and Asian Americans, as well as about Minnesota and, indeed, about Americanness. Mu Daiko's mixed company provides myriad examples of the expansive ways in which Asian America can be performed through taiko.

REPERTOIRE AND SCENARIO: PERFORMING EMBODIED KNOWLEDGE

During my time with Mu Daiko, I performed in countless outreach performances. The majority of these took place in the Twin Cities area, but many of them took me to greater Minnesota and into Wisconsin, Iowa, and the Dakotas. Preparing for these performances was usually quite simple: I had a tote bag dedicated to my outreach gear into which I placed my black tabi, a bright blue happi coat folded into a neat square, my hachimaki, a water bottle, and a smaller drawstring bag containing several pairs of different-sized bachi. While on occasion we performed five-person programs, typical outreach gigs were designed for three performers. We would meet at the Mu Daiko rehearsal space to load up the vehicle, usually Iris's Honda CRV or Rick's minivan. We had developed a formula for fitting all the equipment and performers into a single vehicle: one seat folded down, another pushed forward a notch, and stands and bags slid between the drums. Once we arrived, we would take it all out again and roll our drums, always on wheeled stands, through loading docks, into back entrances, or across parking lots to teach our audiences about taiko (see figures 3.3 and 3.4).

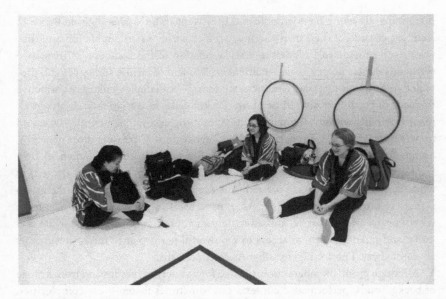

Figure 3.3. Mu Daiko members talk before an outreach performance in Cloquet, Minnesota. Photo by Charissa Uemura. Used with permission.

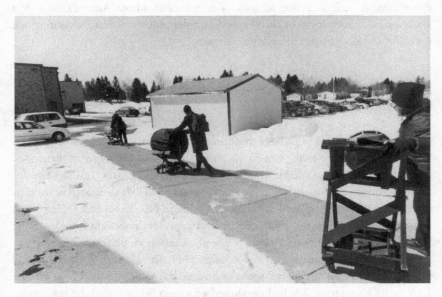

Figure 3.4. Angela Ahlgren, Su-Yoon Ko, and Jennifer Weir roll equipment into an elementary school in Cloquet, Minnesota. Photo by Charissa Uemura. Used with permission.

Mu Daiko members learn, perform, and disseminate embodied knowledge, histories, and values when they play for audiences. Its repertoire includes more than simply the songs the members play; performers produce gestures, facial expressions, and other nonverbal language while on stage, as well as before and after their shows. I am as concerned with thinking about the repertoires of everyday behavior as I am the group's outreach repertoire. In performance circles, "repertoire" most commonly refers to a collection of songs, dances, or plays that a group is prepared to perform. Mu Daiko's repertoire, in this sense, is comprised of taiko pieces, some composed by members of the group and some taught by people outside the group. It typically includes three or four songs, a mixture of "traditional" pieces (that is, arrangements of songs common to many taiko groups) and original compositions by members, interspersed with short lectures and followed by a demonstration in which volunteers from the audience come to the stage to try playing the drums.

I want to think more broadly about repertoire, however, as Diana Taylor does when she uses it to consider how archives and repertoires transmit cultural memory. Repertoires work in tandem with archives, which are thought to be stable and authoritative, based as they are on texts. Repertoire "enacts embodied memory" and "requires presence"; that is, people transmit embodied memory by performing actions. Programs and videotapes of past Mu Daiko performances form part of its archive, but the repertoire itself—the pieces its members can play and which are stored in archives—lives in the bodies of the performers and can be deployed at any time. Repertoires, Taylor claims, "reconstitute themselves, transmitting communal memories, histories, and values from one group/generation to the next. Embodied and performed acts generate, record, and transmit knowledge."[31] It may be useful, for example, to think about San Jose Taiko's "Ei Ja Nai Ka?" as part of a repertoire that generates and transmits knowledge about Japanese American history and pre-internment labor through embodied participation. But any physical practice, from ballet to capoeira to American football, constitutes a repertoire of embodied knowledge that regenerates values, collective histories, and meanings (new or old) each time it is performed.

If "repertoire" names a repository of embodied performances, a set of possible acts to be performed, then each group member has their own personal repertoire, too: not just of Mu Daiko pieces they know, but also partly scripted, memorized, or improvised speeches that they deliver between songs (explaining the names of the drums and how are they made, a brief history of taiko in Japan and North America, or teaching the first phrase of "Matsuri") when in an outreach scenario. More to the point, I ask what repertoire is available to individual performers in enacting interpersonal scenarios beyond the stage: answering questions such as "How long have you been playing? Is it very difficult to learn?" or smiling politely through questions such as "Do you speak English?" or "Where are you from?" As I demonstrate, spectators have their own repertoires, too, embodied knowledge they may have learned not in a studio but at home, in school, or on the playground, consciously or not.

These repertoires of songs, lectures, and everyday behavior are deployed in scenarios, semi-scripted scenes that become familiar by repetition. What might outreach scenarios reveal about Minnesota's racial landscape? About performing Asian America in the Midwest? How might Mu Daiko's performances alternately challenge and affirm received ideas about the Midwest? In a move to consider the embodied dimensions of cultural memory, Taylor invokes scenarios as a gestural counterpart to texts and archives. Because they are enacted physically (repertoire), scenarios exceed textual concerns such as narrative and plot to encompass "milieu and corporeal behaviors such as gestures, attitudes, and tones not reducible to language."[32] I am interested in what cultural values, histories, and meanings are transmitted through outreach scenarios, particularly those that take place off-stage, before and after staged performances, between audiences and performers. Such encounters are constituted by familiar dialogue, embodied repertoires, and backdrops that, taken together, carry with them knowledge, power, and expectations. Taylor writes about "scenarios of discovery," scenes that place the colonized other in the purview of the colonial state. Such scenarios, she writes, "have become so normalized as to transmit values and fantasies without calling attention to itself as a 'conscious' performance."[33] Whereas Taylor uses scenarios of discovery to understand colonial encounters between European explorers and indigenous peoples in the Americas, I adopt the term to describe encounters between taiko performers and audiences in the context of American Orientalism and multiculturalism at the turn of the twenty-first century.

Presentations of art forms such as taiko—that is, forms that might be categorized as world music, ethnic dance, or non-Western performance—often play out in predictable ways, in their own scenarios of discovery. Each performance can unfold in any number of ways, but expectations based on previous iterations teach audiences how to behave. Cultural festivals and international expositions, or World's Fairs, have laid groundwork that teaches (especially) white audiences to approach Asian American performers as foreign and exotic. Mu Daiko's outreach costumes, which include Japanese workers' garments, as well as publicity materials that emphasize taiko's "ancient" roots, can contribute to such a reading.[34]

One scenario goes like this: As we pack up our drums after a performance, a white man approaches and begins speaking in stilted Japanese to one of our Asian American performers. Any of them can only reply, "I don't speak Japanese." (At that time, the only member of Mu Daiko who spoke Japanese fluently was Rachel, a white woman from Minnesota.) Another scenario might unfold this way: I am performing alongside two Japanese American women, and each of us has delivered one of the lecture segments into a microphone between numbers. After the performance, an audience member approaches me and asks if my co-performers speak English, despite the fact that both of them spoke English during the performance. In another instance, a young white man wearing a wide cotton headband in the style of a martial arts uniform approaches one of Mu Daiko's Korean American members as we pack up our drums and tries to engage her in conversation about his enthusiasm for all things Japanese.[35] The first two scenarios reveal the pervasive assumption that Asians are perpetual foreigners, always newly arrived from elsewhere, even when they speak English, possibly with a Minnesota accent. The third scenario further reveals the exotic appeal of taiko and its performers for some audience members whose enthusiasm for Japanese culture tends toward the Asiaphilic. In other instances spectators' reactions to white group members reveal their expectations of Asian authenticity, an issue I explore in more depth in Chapter 4.

Yet scenarios of discovery within taiko performance are not limited to an Orientalist framework; they can play out in other ways. In Taylor's framing, because these scenarios are part of an embodied repertoire, not a fixed archive, they harbor the possibility of change. "The body," she writes, "has space to maneuver because it is not scripted."[36] Indeed, as I demonstrate here, although Orientalism is often woven into taiko outreach, it is just one part of a complex scenario that takes place in Mu Daiko's performances because taiko players are aware of and responsive to this potential. From a performer's perspective, Mu Daiko's outreach shows are often the simplest performances to carry out because they are low-tech (requiring only a microphone for speaking segments), include familiar repertoire (most of them are the first pieces students learn in taiko classes), and operate on a basic format with which all performers become familiar. As member Jeff Ellsworth describes it, "You roll in, you play, you roll out."[37] Because the structure of each performance, including the ways drums are packed and transported, is relatively set, it can become routine. The performance material is predictable enough that several performers noted that they use outreach as an opportunity to experiment with their own playing, either by trying out a new solo or experimenting with new techniques as they play. After mentioning the routine aspects of outreach, Ellsworth stated in the same breath that "it's something different every time." Some performances become legendary: performing barefoot in a field while turkeys roamed the ground and apples fell from trees overhead; playing in a maintenance closet at the Mall of America; or being invited to play in libraries only to be shushed. The unpredictability of each performance context requires players to improvise, both on and off-stage: just as they adjust their spacing and choreography to fit onto the cramped stages and slippery floors of such nontheatrical spaces as cafeterias and gymnasiums (or grass, gravel, and pavement for outdoor performances), performers must also improvise responses to spectators' questions and clients' expectations, often negotiating issues of race, gender, and national identity.

An outreach performance that I attended demonstrates how the fleshy, real-time encounter of the outreach scenario, coupled with its less formal structure and setting, produces meanings and histories without seeming to do anything at all. On June 20, 2009, I accompanied a trio of Mu Daiko members to an event hosted by a nonprofit organization called Honoring Women Worldwide, which is focused on developing women's leadership across cultures.[38]

We arrived at the event, held in the Women's Suffrage Memorial Garden on the lush green grass that slopes gently toward the state capitol in St. Paul. Outreach director Susie Kuniyoshi had asked three women—Iris Shiraishi, Heather Jeche, and Eileen Ho—to play the gig, since it was a women's event. As we began to unload the drums, a large group of women, at least one-third of whom were women of color, mingled near the rows of chairs and dais set up on the grass. The coordinator of the event asked us to set up our equipment on the sidewalk, which would provide more stability for the drums but which also had the unfortunate effect of sidelining the performance when there was ample room near the dais. Mu Daiko's role in the event was to capture people's attention with their drumming before the event formally began.

As the players dressed and warmed up for their performance, a white woman, perhaps in her sixties or seventies, approached and told us that she'd seen us perform at another event. "I love your little costumes," she said. The performers smiled and thanked her, but the belittling tone of the comment did not escape their notice. When the three Mu Daiko women were signaled to begin their performance, I took a seat on a low stone wall at the edge of the garden; the seats set up for the event did not face in a direction that allowed attendees to see the players. The drummers began the formal *oroshi*, or introductory crescendo beats, for the first song, "Mu Shu." Taiko often is used to kick off events, since its sonic and kinesthetic hugeness is difficult to ignore. Yet on that day, the drummers had trouble capturing the audience's attention. Perhaps playing outside on a humid day loosened the drumheads and dampened the sound, or perhaps the performers' position off to the side rather than on the grass in front of the audience made it difficult for them to pay attention. As Mu Daiko played, the audience continued to mingle and talk. At one point an entire family walked right through the playing area, between the drummers as they played, though there was ample room in which to walk around them. All three performers' smiles widened when this happened: they were amused or annoyed, but they remained unflappable. Another woman walked up to Iris in the middle of a song and tried to talk to her as she played the *shime*. Iris flashed me a "this is so weird" smile but she kept the beat steady. Perhaps this will become one of those legendary gigs ("Remember the time . . . ?"). The crowd didn't truly pay attention to the performance until the third and final song, "Ni Dan," an intricately choreographed piece that requires performers to whirl around and between drums (see figure 3.5). As we packed up the drums, the main event at Honoring Women Worldwide began in earnest.

As we drove back to the Mu Daiko rehearsal space after the outreach, our conversation combined practical considerations with theorizing of the gender politics inherent in the event. The members commented on the audience's behavior and the unfortunate way in which an event meant to honor women had rendered three women performers peripheral, both by asking them to play on the edges of the event space and by not making their performance a formal part of the program lineup. Placing them on the sidelines enabled audience members to either ignore them completely or to invade their performance space as they played. They were more of a curiosity than a group of women to be honored along with those involved in the event.

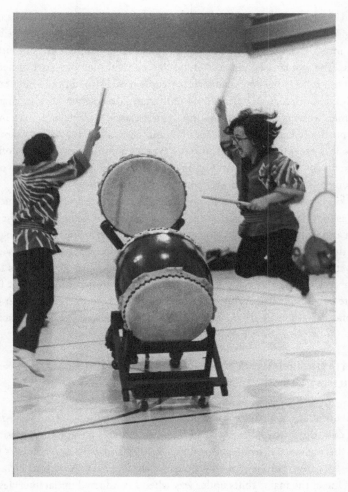

Figure 3.5. Su-Yoon Ko and Jennifer Weir play Mu Daiko's outreach arrangement of "Ni Dan" in Cloquet, Minnesota. Photo by Charissa Uemura. Used with permission.

As performers, they improvised by adjusting to playing on a sidewalk and continuing to play the drums while people walked perilously close to them during the performance. But they also improvised responses to audience members before and after the performance. When the woman said, "I love your little costumes," the performers responded politely. Perhaps they even tried to give her more information about the costumes (modeled after workers' attire) or what they are called (happi coats, obi, and hachimaki). She had been friendly, yet her calling the costumes "little" was at odds with the ways taiko is so often experienced as large, empowering, and even overpowering in its sonic and visual effects. In this scenario a white woman spoke to a group of Asian American women who in mere moments would be ferociously beating the drums. Yet her comment literally belittled the costumes, and by extension, the women wearing them. It is difficult to imagine the same comment being directed at white or male performers because it plays into a racialized and feminized image of Asian women as diminutive and doll-like. The woman's behavior is embodied cultural memory, part of her repertoire, and it reflects the way many white people have learned how to interact with and think about Asian people. Seeing utilitarian Japanese worker's garments and the women wearing them as little supports the classic Orientalist binary in which Asia is positioned as childlike, decorative, and objectified. I give this example not because it is exceptional but because the type of comment the woman offered is familiar: meant as a compliment but unable to avoid the entrenched view of Asian costuming or Asian American women as anything but little or quaint.

The kinds of scenarios I have described briefly here reveal as much about the audience as they do about the performers. Asian Americans being asked if they speak English and white performers being asked if their co-performers speak English are part of the repertoire of American Orientalism in which Asian Americans are seen as perpetually foreign and unfamiliar, or in Karen Shimakawa's terms, as the "national abject," always outside of or constituting the limits of the nation. Perhaps these are encounters that Asian American taiko players across North America have experienced, but these particular scenarios reflect Minnesota's racial landscape.

NEGOTIATING IDENTITY AND PERFORMING EMOTIONAL LABOR

As a racially mixed company of taiko players tied to Minnesota's first Asian American theater company, Mu Daiko itself has negotiated issues of race and identity, both among themselves and while performing. In 2009 and 2010 the members were in the midst of conversations about the group's relation to Asian American social justice issues. One of the major shifts under way when I conducted initial interviews with Mu Daiko members was the receipt of a large grant from Asian American Pacific Islanders in Philanthropy (AAPIP), which had a number of stipulations attached.[39] One way in which Mu qualified for the grant was by arguing that issues of social justice were inherent in the company's activities, if not explicitly stated in its mission at the time. Mu Performing Arts as a whole was thus revising how it articulated its mission via mainstage plays, taiko concerts, and outreach performance. Accordingly, Mu Daiko leaders and members were negotiating the group's Asian Americanness through decisions about marketing, casting, and scripting of outreach at a time when they sought to foreground social justice as a key facet of the company.

Rick Shiomi had been the artistic director of the theater side (since 1993) and the taiko side (since 1997). Shiomi spoke candidly about how issues of race and social justice were affecting Mu Daiko when I asked about the direction of the company, particularly as it related to the AAPIP grant. He explained that long before he founded the taiko group, he had been working with social justice issues in theater, particularly by creating opportunities for underrepresented Asian American theater artists. "All of my work," he told me, "was about social, cultural history and social justice and those kinds of issues within theater. . . . it's already inherent in the work that we do."[40] In other words, the plays Mu produces often have issues of social justice wound into them, even if they are not overtly about politics.

When I began with Mu Daiko, the group's ties to Asian American cultural politics seemed implicit in its affiliation with Theater Mu, but they were not made an explicit part of group membership. Although taiko in North America emerged from an era of Asian American social justice activism, Mu Daiko's engagement with the subject is less obvious. Addressing these issues within Mu Performing Arts "changes more in taiko than in theater," Shiomi said, because

> [i]n theatre, you have all these Asian American actors. You don't have to explain to them the issues they face as Asian American actors because every time they go audition at another company, they realize: "They're not looking at us because we're Asian American. They don't think we're any good or that we're going to fit into this situation." . . . [A]ctors talk about issues. But taiko players don't do that, taiko players don't talk about discrimination. Most of them are not Asian American anyway, and so they're not thinking in those terms. So now [Mu Daiko has] gone ten years with all that happening and nobody ever talked about it. So now we're starting to talk about it.[41]

Looking at Mu Daiko's evolution as a group whose initial membership was comprised entirely of Asian American theater artists to one whose membership has only a few people who do theater work, it makes sense that values that were implicit in the beginning would shift along with the group's composition. In his comments, Shiomi essentialized differences between actors and taiko players to make the point that Asian American actors, whose livelihood depends on being selected for specific roles, are especially familiar with not only rejection based on race (or producers' racist preferences) but also a long history of Orientalist and degrading roles being the only ones available to them. What Shiomi suggested is that Asian American actors are aware that what they are doing is inherently political. Indeed, they have been talking about discrimination since the 1960s, when some of the first protests over unfair casting practices were staged in New York and the first Asian American theater companies were founded, the same cultural-political milieu from which the first taiko groups emerged.[42]

Of course, many taiko players do talk about and speak out against racism. Those who founded the first North American taiko groups in the 1960s and 1970s—most of them Asian Americans—certainly understood the relation between performance and racial representation. As the remainder of the chapter demonstrates, Mu Daiko members are, indeed, aware of issues that face Asian Americans on- and off-stage. But Shiomi's comment indicated that some members felt excluded or at least anxious about how they would fit into a group with a more explicit focus on Asian American social justice issues.

Shiomi's past as a community organizer in Vancouver in the late 1970s and his continuing work developing Asian American theater artists aligns him with the ideals of the Asian American movement. His ideas thus also reflect the philosophy of San Jose Taiko, which he described as having "a deliberate cultural intentionality and Asian American intentionality." Although San Jose Taiko's audition process includes readings and discussion about the group's origins in an era of Asian American activism, neither it nor Mu Daiko limits membership to Asian Americans. To do so, Shiomi said, would be antithetical to his work with Seiichi Tanaka of San Francisco Taiko Dojo, a man and group that have maintained a decidedly integrationist philosophy in terms of teaching taiko: "Tanaka-sensei's school is he says, 'Anyone that wants to play taiko, wants to learn taiko, wants to study with me I'll teach them. I don't care if they're green, blue, yellow, or black, whatever.' And [Tanaka] wants everyone in America to play taiko and everyone in America to love taiko."[43] Rick's characterization of Tanaka's philosophy reflected Tanaka's oft-cited goal to make taiko as familiar to Americans as sushi and karate.[44] As an art form that emerged from Asian American experiences, as well as from Japan, taiko "in its most basic forms" showcases performance "from the Asian American experience." Apart from Shiomi's background in Asian American activism and theater, Mu Daiko has also operated in such a way that anyone, regardless of racial identity, can participate. "But," he said, "could I imagine a group where there were no Asian Americans in it? I don't think so."[45] Here, his "I don't think so" is a statement not of indecision but of certainty. That is, the way he uttered "I don't think so" sounds more like, "Not on your life." It did not mean that he had not yet fully considered a Mu Daiko without Asian Americans; it is confirmation that he had imagined it, and it was not acceptable.

Mu Daiko was, after all, part of a theater company whose mission is to produce works that address Asian American issues in some significant way, and Mu Daiko outreach performances staffed entirely with white players can make it seem as though it is a group without Asian Americans. These issues were familiar to Susie Kuniyoshi in her role as outreach director. When asked to book performances whose purpose was to "provide role modeling," she said, "I [had] to try really hard to get a group together that has at least one Asian person in it." It may seem a simple task in a group one-half of whose members generally are Asian Americans, but she needed to balance people's availability as well as aspects of their identities. Regarding the need to meet the clients' expectations, she said, "I've had complaints afterwards from people who said, you know, 'We brought you in as, to show a Japanese group, and why were all the people white?'"

Kuniyoshi recalled the time one client remarked, "What a world we live in when we celebrate Chinese New Year by bringing in a Japanese drumming group of all white people." In fact, Gregg Amundsen and Al Zdrazil both mentioned the same outreach performance to me in my interviews with them, and Susie, Gregg, and Al reminded me that I'd been one of the players. My memories of this particular performance are vague at best, but I remember feeling self-conscious in moments when

I was in outreach performances where all three players were white. Gregg, on the other hand, felt differently, telling me, "I've never been uncomfortable performing in those contexts. I sometimes wonder if the people who are booking this—I mean, I look at it as, I'm being hired to do this job, I'll just go out and do it. Um, I just wonder . . . it's like, 'Is this what you had planned on?' "[46] Having white performers is not unique to Mu Daiko, but the group's affiliation with Theater Mu, combined with clients' motives for hiring the group, creates an undesirable situation when white performers act as Asian American role models. Given that the matter of white artists appropriating Asian forms and the phenomenon dubbed "whitewashing," in which roles written for Asians are recast with white actors, are issues that Theater Mu was created to critique and resist, having an all-white Mu Daiko outreach group does not align with the mission of the company.

Asian American performers' experiences of participating in Mu Daiko outreach reveal ambivalence about their roles as taiko players in the Midwest. "Ambivalence" typically refers to holding multiple or contradictory feelings at the same time. Here, I use the term to describe feelings, but also to point to a cultural position in the sense that these players' ambivalence is informed by a number of discourses that precede any one person's experience of taiko. All three of the Asian American women I interviewed mentioned the potential for positive role modeling (especially for girls and Asian Americans), while acknowledging that outreach sometimes requires the emotional labor of maintaining politeness while fielding racist commentary. Heewon Lee, for example, mentioned that she appreciated being a person of color performing in places with very few Asians. In those situations, she said, "you see [Asian or other students of color] and you see how excited they are to see you on stage, [and] it does make a really big difference. You're like, 'Oh, I'm playing for you.' " On the other hand, she said taiko "has the danger of being exoticized. So I always kind of think about that double-edged sword." For example, when taiko is treated as side entertainment in outreach rather than the main event, she often felt like "the exotic Asian hired help," particularly when the performance took place in a largely white business environment.[47] These contexts can reinforce the notion that Mu Daiko performers are on display, being continually discovered and gazed upon by white spectators.

Lee critiqued Mu Daiko's standard outreach scenario, particularly the Japanese costumes and the absence of much contextualizing information about Asian American genealogies of taiko, for aiding such Orientalist readings. During my membership and field work with Mu Daiko, it was usual to repeat commonly accepted ideas about taiko's early history, which can reinforce false notions of taiko as an ancient art form and of Japan as firmly located in the distant past. For example, we would often relate the fact that taiko drums have been used for many centuries in Japan, along with the less well-substantiated claims that taiko were used in harvest festivals and battles and even used as a way to demarcate the boundaries of villages. Rehearsing a history of a form rooted in an ancient and rural past obscures the twentieth-century history of taiko, which is a product of the 1950s and also, primarily, of the urban performance scene in Tokyo.[48] Mu performers may also discuss Mu Daiko's connection to San Francisco Taiko Dojo by noting that Rick Shiomi had studied with Seiichi Tanaka, who brought taiko from Japan to California. Though true, this history oversimplifies the genealogy of taiko's development in North America and obscures taiko's connections to Asian American movement politics, not to mention the presence of women as players and leaders. Of course, the time constraints and the attention span of the audience (particularly when it includes children) prevent us from relating more complex genealogies of taiko. My goal is not to criticize the Mu Daiko outreach scripts but to point to the ways we as performers sometimes reinforce, rather than unsettle, audience's tendencies toward Orientalist views of taiko.[49] Thus, even when Mu Daiko members have the opportunity to narrate taiko history, the scripts can reinforce Heewon Lee's observation that taiko outreach is haunted by past Orientalist displays and performances.[50] As Taylor explains, scenarios are "never for the first time, and never for the last," but "constantly reactivated in the now of performance."[51]

The way performers react to feeling exoticized or stigmatized varies, too. In our interview, Jennifer Weir discussed offstage encounters with audience members whose racism unsettled her. She noted that audience remarks

> reveal so many of the things that frustrate you as a person of color, as an Asian American . . . stupid, racist, bizarre comments. And you kind of shake your head and try to laugh them off or sort of be kindly educating in the process. But there's always that element out there, and you never kind of know when it will hit you, and if it will amuse you or enrage you at any given moment.[52]

Rather than focusing on the Orientalist potential within taiko performance, Weir highlighted the everyday nature of racist encounters for Asian Americans and other people of color. Such experiences are, perhaps, exacerbated by the very public performances intended to correct the attitudes revealed in those encounters. Her words also pointed to the emotional labor required of performers hired out as representatives of a theater company. During our interview, Weir laughed about these experiences as she noted that sometimes people's ignorant questions reflect their "best intentions even if they're saying something really offensive and stupid." As if reminding herself, she told me that she, too, hadn't always been self-aware about "race or self or culture or queerness" when she was younger and so was typically willing to "give [people] a little slack." Having grown up as a Korean adoptee raised by white parents in the geographically remote city of Minot, North Dakota, understanding her own race and sexuality was a gradual process. Although racist comments are both commonplace and potentially enraging, Weir acknowledged the processual nature of acquiring knowledge about her own identity, let alone someone else's.

Iris Shiraishi similarly expressed her critique of audience racism with equanimity. When I asked if she had experienced racism during outreach performances, she recalled that she, Rachel Gorton, and Su-Yoon Ko had gone on a short tour in mostly rural areas of Minnesota. "I just remember a couple of times when we walked into the cafes, and people would just go [she mimes a wide-eyed stare and then laughs]. Thank god for Rachel." Rachel was the only white woman on the tour, and Iris's mention of her clearly indicated that Rachel's presence eased some of the nervousness she'd felt. She continued, "Between [Su-Yoon] and me . . . we kind of like increased the Asian population by one hundred percent . . . those were not comfortable experiences."[53] Though she discussed this topic with me in a lighthearted way, joking about Rachel's being a buffer between them and the towns' white populations, her anecdote points to real issues of safety and the ways performers of color—even those doing seemingly uncontroversial taiko outreach performance—put their bodies on the line when they perform and travel to unfamiliar areas (or rather, areas in which they are regarded as unfamiliar).

Shiraishi also pointed out that her outreach experiences were mostly positive and that, although she did field ignorant comments, "You know they're not saying it out of racism and you know they're not saying it out of meanness or cruelty. It's just because they don't know." The most common question of this sort, she said, was being asked whether she spoke English. Shiraishi and Weir both attribute audiences' questions about race to ignorance or lacking knowledge that they may yet acquire. Part of the reason may have to do with their knowledge that part of the goal of outreach performance is to educate audiences. It is also possible that Asian American Mu Daiko members downplay their own perceptions of audience racism because, as Kim Park Nelson points out in *Invisible Asians*, acknowledging racism is seldom rewarded in public culture.[54]

Heewon Lee's view concerning the innocence of racist comments was somewhat different. "With racism," she said, "it's not the overt stuff, it's the really nice, well-intentioned people coming to say these ridiculous things that they don't even realize the privilege and they don't even realize, you know, what system makes it okay for them to say that." Although Lee was not speaking of any specific instance, her comment resonated with the situation the outreach group faced at the Honoring Women Worldwide event, when a white woman did not seem to understand the condescension inherent in her comment about little costumes. Lee continued, "And being on the job, you can't really say, you know, 'f--- you' or 'no way.' You just have to sort of do your best to be diplomatic and kind of ease out of it." Lee's comments, as well as Weir's choice to sometimes respond in a "kindly educating" way, point beyond the racist (and in this case, also sexist) sentiment that players may face to the ways racial (and gender and sexual) minorities are often expected to either dismiss as unintentional or kindly correct offensive language directed at them. Lee's remarks showed that she viewed "ridiculous things" people say as racist, regardless of their intention. Yet as a representative of Mu Daiko and as a woman of color in a majority white culture, she cannot always respond in the way she might want to.

These examples demonstrate that outreach performance requires people of color to expend emotional labor using a limited repertoire of performative gestures, facial expressions, and language that are deemed appropriate to not only professional situations, but white culture. Arlie Hochschild, in her influential study of flight attendants in the 1980s, defines "emotional labor" as "the management of feeling to create a publicly observable facial and bodily display," especially that which is sold for wages.[55] Building on Hochschild's (and others') work, Louwanda Evans and Wendy Leo Moore argue that more emotional labor is required of people of color working within white institutions. They write, "[E]ven as people of color are forced to negotiate systematic racial micro-aggressions that objectify and other them . . . their responses are constrained" because dominant racial logics deny the existence of racism.[56] In many cases, Mu Daiko members are performing within white institutions, and when they are not actually in institutional settings, they are navigating geographies that are white-dominated. Outreach performance requires emotional labor, which is racialized and gendered, and it also yokes the performers' taiko repertoire with their own and their audience's repertoire of racial etiquette. As performers and representatives of Mu Daiko and Mu Performing Arts, they also are aware that it would seem inappropriate to respond angrily or coldly in such situations. While the scenario may require them to improvise, they understand the repertoire of choices to be limited: smiling, polite, and diplomatic responses are the available options. Weir stated that her potential emotional responses ranged from amusement to rage, but her appropriate outward responses were limited to laughter or a "kindly educating" response of some kind. Similarly, Lee described diplomacy as the socially acceptable outward response to racist comments, even though her impulse might be to respond with anger. The repertoire of responses available to Mu Daiko members, especially women of color, in outreach scenarios is limited not only because they are on the job but also because moderating responses to racist encounters is a survival strategy for people of color. As Sarah Ahmed points out in her book *Living a Feminist Life*, "When you expose a problem you pose a problem."[57] In other words, were Mu Daiko members to point out the racism inherent in their spectators' questions, they themselves would be seen as creating a problem, since mainstream views dictate that racism does not exist. Such instances of racial innocence in the context of performing in Minnesota are the topic of the following section.

PERFORMING RACIAL INNOCENCE

If I may return to the snow globe with which I opened the chapter, it seems that Minnesota's reputation as monolithically white seldom leaves room for discussions of racism. Yet the experiences of Mu Daiko members demonstrate that it exists on a number of levels. In this section I examine the encounters that Susie Kuniyoshi had when she toured northern Minnesota and Wisconsin schools as a flutist in an orchestra in the decade just before Mu Daiko was founded. In my interview with her, Kuniyoshi narrated vivid recollections of being the target of racism during these tours. Although her recollections were not about Mu Daiko outreach, her experiences provide context for the rural areas of the region. I had known Susie for about ten years when I interviewed her in June 2009. Not only had we performed in Mu Daiko together, but we had also worked together as staff members for Mu Performing Arts. Some taiko players were reluctant to discuss race and racism with me, even when I asked about it specifically. Susie, by contrast, described her early years in Minnesota as rife with instances of racism and feelings of not belonging.

Susie was born in Hilo, Hawai'i, and had come to Minnesota from the East coast, where she had studied music at Ithaca College and then the Boston Conservatory. Moving to the mainland had in itself brought "major culture shock," but moving several years later to Duluth, a relatively isolated northern Minnesota city of approximately ninety thousand people, was another one, because, she said, "When I got to Duluth it was completely—[she looked at me] well, everybody looks like you. It was completely blonde, Scandinavian, Germanic population up there when I moved there." I knew what she meant because I grew up in Cloquet, Minnesota, thirty minutes from Duluth, and my whiteness, Finnish heritage, and Swedish-derived surname have always meant that I blend in there.

Susie described two examples of the kinds of racist encounters she experienced in northern Minnesota and northern Wisconsin. In one instance, a group of six or seven blond girls surrounded her in a bathroom and stared at her. When I asked if they'd done anything beyond stare, she said, "They were just intimidating me." The presence of a group of white girls surrounding a lone Japanese American woman created a threatening scenario; their powerful choreography of surrounding and focusing their collective gaze on Susie required no words to communicate its meaning.

In order to describe the other incident, I share an excerpt from the interview transcript to prioritize her telling of it and also to reflect on my own reactions to the telling. Rather than focus only on her narrative, I also highlight the scenario of our interview and, in particular, my role as a white interlocutor in order to examine further the very racial innocence I critiqued earlier.

SK: I remember I was playing in the UWS [University of Wisconsin at Superior, near Duluth] faculty woodwind quintet up there, and we did a tour of Wisconsin, and I remember when we arrived at the school in Ashland [on the northern border of Wisconsin, about seventy miles east of Duluth], and we were walking through the hallways to go to the room where we were going to perform . . . all of a sudden, these boys started following me down the hallway and making machine gun sounds.

AA: Oh, wow.

SK: They were, yeah, they were like, you know, miming—

AA: Yeah.

SK: -—the shooting.

AA: Was that, like, a Vietnam War kind of reference or something?

SK: I think so.

AA: It's just so horrible.

SK: Yeah, it's just, yeah, "shoot the gooks" kind of thing. Because when I was in Duluth, a lot of times, I would get gook comments.

AA: Really.

SK: Yeah.

AA: That's really fascinating.

SK: Yeah.

AA: It just doesn't seem—

SK: It was very, I did not like touring the schools. I was very uncomfortable touring the schools because of incidents like that and having to go through stuff like that.

Our dialogue captures the kinds of racist encounters that Susie experienced in Minnesota as an Asian American artist, as well as my sense of awe ("wow," "horrible," "fascinating") and outright disbelief ("It just doesn't seem—") at such overt acts of racism. Reading the transcript several years later, I wondered what the rest of my sentence would have been: "It just doesn't seem—*like something a Minnesotan would do?—like children would know the racist repertoire of "shooting a gook"?—like racist slurs would live on decades after a war has ended?*" Any of these possible reactions now seems wildly naïve on my part: Minnesotans are often racist, and not only in the asking of ignorant questions; the children she spoke of certainly learned racist language and gestures at a young age; and racial slurs endure long after their initial use. Yet I was clearly surprised during this interview. On one hand, as she acknowledged, my experience of Minnesota was quite different because I was never a target of racism when I lived there. On the other hand, part of my reaction also came from the boys' use of a machine-gun gesture and Susie's admission that she had frequently been called a gook, a slur I incorrectly associated exclusively with the war in Vietnam.

The story she shared surprised me, but it shouldn't have. As a scholar of race and performance I needed reminding that racial slurs and images outlast their original usage and that they remain flexible and durable. The term "gook," according to David Roediger, had been used to identify and dehumanize a range of nonwhite others long before it became associated specifically with Asians, the Vietnam War only a late stop in a linguistic history that began in the late nineteenth century. An Americanism, "gook" has been used to target Haitians, Filipinos, Arabs, Koreans, and Vietnamese. The term, Roediger writes, was used widely and casually in print to describe Asians, most starkly perhaps in 1969, when the reporter Robert Kaiser claimed, "The only good gook, it is said again and again on US bases throughout Vietnam, is a dead gook."[58] Roediger continues, "The stark dehumanization of enemies in such a line reminds us that racism is not only a way to motivate fighters in wars of aggression but also that militarism has helped to foster racism."[59] In 2000, Senator John McCain publicly used—and stood by his right to use—the term with little political consequence.[60] That racism is so deeply linked to military conflicts and an us-versus-them mentality is part of what allows people such as McCain to (unjustly) defend his use of a racial slur in a public forum and what allows children in a rural Midwestern school to mimic shooting an adult woman and educator with machine guns.

Notice that the children did not *call* Susie a gook. They mimed shooting her. We know what it looks like, the convulsive, outstretched arms spraying imaginary bullets across a wide target. They uttered not words but machine-gun noises. We know what they sound like, too. These performances are part of a repertoire that complements the archival—the textual and documented—history of anti-Asian racism. As Robin Bernstein brilliantly demonstrates, in the nineteenth century white children routinely and wantonly brutalized black dolls, which, she argues, were crafted specifically as alternatives to delicate white dolls to withstand and invite such violence, since it was widely believed that black children could not experience pain. Because white children's violence toward the dolls was collective—that is, it was enacted with other children and described in widely circulated publications—white children became not simply "repositories and reflectors of racist culture; they were its co-producers."[61] When the boys mimed shooting Susie with machine guns, they performed and re-produced a scenario of racial violence familiar from decades' worth of literature, film, popular culture, and children's war play, repertoire that clearly lived on long after the war in Vietnam. We might, in fact, think of this repertoire as the counterpart to San Jose Taiko's "Ei Ja Nai Ka?"—an embodied history that continues to be danced and performed into being (see Chapter 2). Whereas that piece invites participants to co-perform Asian American histories that have been left out of U.S. historical narratives, this "shoot the gook" child's play performs and reproduces dominant narratives of exclusion and eradication of Asians from the country.

My reaction to the racist encounters that Susie related in the interview dovetails with what author David Mura writes about Minnesota and racism. Despite increasing media attention to racial violence and social disparities in the state, he argues, Minnesotans prefer to avoid discussions of racism. Whites there "like to think of themselves as nice people."[62] Although a central topic of my interview with Susie had been race, this particular incident produced disbelief, if momentary. It is tempting to apply the label "Minnesota Nice" to several of the encounters I have related in this chapter. The phrase belies its own double-edged nature, as the niceness also comes with aloofness, especially toward those who are outsiders for one reason or another. Such a construct, however, allows racism to be excused or dismissed as ignorance. As Bernstein writes, "Racial innocence is a form of deflection, a not-knowing or obliviousness that can be made politically useful."[63] Minnesota Nice, then, is a repertoire that allows "nice" white Minnesotans to play out racist scenarios while deflecting charges of racism. We might also see not only the children's acts of racist intimidation, but also the white woman's admiration of Mu Daiko's little costumes and spectators' inquiries about performers' English-speaking abilities, as part of a repertoire of Midwestern racial innocence. The stakes of interrupting this repertoire are high, since it covers countless acts of racial violence.[64]

When Mu Daiko members go out into the Twin Cities, greater Minnesota, and other Midwestern states as representatives of Mu Performing Arts, they perform Asian America. Whether or not each player is Asian American, with their corporeal presence onstage playing Japanese drums (albeit ones made in Minnesota), representing an Asian American performing arts company, they co-constitute Asian American performance. As I have demonstrated, this performance happens at the level of a staged concert and as a series of improvised scenarios between audience and performers in a variety of settings. In the following section I explore the ways in which outreach performance exceeds the scripted scenarios and expands the ways Asian Americanness and Minnesotanness are performed and contested.

SCENARIOS OF RECOGNITION: KOREAN ADOPTEES AND TAIKO

If Mu Daiko outreach performances reveal the racial logic that renders Asian Americans perpetual foreigners or objects of exoticism, they also reveal the complexity and multiplicity within Minnesota's Asian American communities. As I mentioned above, the group has included people of Japanese, Chinese, Korean, Indian, Indonesian, and European descent. Several of Mu Daiko's members have been Korean American adoptees, including (but not limited to) three interviewed for this study. Although Asian Americans comprise a relatively small percentage of the state's overall population, "Minnesota is home to the largest per capita population of Korean adoptees in the United States," according to American studies scholar Kim Park Nelson.[65] Furthermore, they make up one-half of the Korean American population of the state.[66] In her study of their experiences, Park Nelson illustrates these figures in the language of the state's lore, writing, "The population of Korean American adoptees in the state of Minnesota, estimated to be between ten thousand and fifteen thousand, suggests a half-joking parallel with the state motto, 'The Land of 10,000 Lakes.' In fact, there are about fifteen thousand lakes in Minnesota, so it would be accurate to say that there is indeed a Korean adoptee for every lake."[67] Nonetheless, the state's relatively small Asian American population has resulted in many adoptees' reporting "extreme racial isolation" in their lives.[68] And because they are racial minorities raised in mostly white families, many Korean adoptees also report "a profound sense of racial in-betweenness."[69] Such experiences, along with a range of adoptee voices and perspectives, have been represented in Mu's theatrical productions since the company's inception, and Korean adoptees work with Mu Performing Arts as theater and taiko artists and as administrators.[70]

In what follows, I explore the outreach scenarios embedded in the interviews and artwork of Mu Daiko members who are Korean adoptees. Although my research was not designed with the goal of examining such experiences, the Korean American members I interviewed described their participation in taiko in terms of their identity as adoptees. In the remaining pages of the chapter I analyze an interview with Jennifer Weir, who narrated two encounters that highlight the particularities of being a Korean adoptee taiko player. I end with a close reading of Mu Daiko member Su-Yoon Ko's spoken-word performance "Reaching," which details her ambivalence about being a Korean adoptee performing in Minnesota schools. My analyses depend on the wealth of recent Asian American studies scholarship that centers on transracial and international adoption. These outreach scenarios, then, can be seen not merely as part of Mu Daiko's history but also as part of a larger movement in which activism, scholarship, and cultural production by, for, and about Korean adoptees and other transracial adoptees has flourished. This is significant because historically, studies of adoption have been rather myopically focused on either government policies or the experiences of adoptive parents; recent studies that validate the perspectives of adult adoptees raise myriad issues including intersections between transnational adoption and imperialism, American exceptionalism, and military occupations.[71] My analysis foregrounds the ways the Korean adoptee players theorize their own experiences and shows how their presence challenges received notions of what it means to be Minnesotan and Midwestern.

When I interviewed Jennifer Weir, who was adopted from South Korea and raised in Minot, North Dakota, she recounted two memorable moments of interaction with Korean audience members at outreach performances. The scenarios she described constituted moments in which performer and audience improvised a scenario of discovery in ways that departed from and exceed an American Orientalist framework but which pointed to the historical and cultural place of Korean adoptees within Asian America and within Minnesota. These scenarios complicate notions of what it means to perform Asian America and suggest, as Josephine Lee does, that these experiences of racial isolation "should be thought of as a paradigmatic rather than a peripheral part of Asian American experience."[72]

Responding to a question about outreach performance Weir recalled packing up after an engagement in the small southern Minnesota city of Red Wing and being approached by a young Asian American boy who asked if she was Japanese. She told the boy she was Korean and Weir said, "[H]is face lit up and he said, 'Me, too!'" When the boy ran over to his white father to say, "She's Korean too!" Weir recognized him as (likely) an adopted Korean. "I almost bawled right there," she said.[73] In this scenario, the young boy and Weir recognized each other first as Asian Americans; he (mis)recognized her as Japanese initially and then learned that she was Korean. Weir recognized a familiar racial dynamic, that of a white parent with a Korean, presumably adopted, child. Weir's emotional response, nearly crying, exceeds the scripted outreach scenario in which the performer teaches audience members about the art form, even as it fulfills the promise of "outreach" by reaching out to (or, rather, by being reached by) Asian Americans in greater Minnesota. Here, taiko outreach was more than simple multicultural exchange or Orientalist display. In another situation the boy's question, "Are you Japanese?" may have led to an entirely different sort of encounter, an Orientalist assumption that all Asians look alike. But here the same script forms the basis for a powerful moment of recognition. In this little boy, Weir recognized not just another Asian American or even another Korean adoptee but an entire experience of growing up Asian American in a white family in the Midwest. That she may have been seen as a role model, even momentarily, for this boy echoes other Mu Daiko members' sentiments that role modeling was one of the rewards of outreach.

In Weir's other recollection, she and another Korean adoptee, Heewon Lee, performed not in an idyllic small town, but in the heart of the city. Weir recounted:

> We played on a gravel, empty lot where there was broken glass and dirt over in the Riverside area [of Minneapolis] . . . so it was, you know, very, very diverse community, very, you know, economically challenged. . . . And we played for a festival that they were having, and there just happens to be a housing project there where a lot of retired or elder Korean people live. And so this Korean woman came up to me and Heewon and tried to talk to us in Korean. And both of us, like, it broke our hearts that we couldn't respond to her, you know, or just . . . the fact that she would come and reach out and recognize us as being Korean and want to talk to us and say something, and that we didn't have the ability to even say hello back . . . that was heartbreaking to me on a personal level.[74]

In this scenario Weir and Lee were recognized as Korean, but unlike the young boy being raised in an English-speaking white family, the elderly Korean woman, apparently an immigrant, could not communicate with the two women she recognized as fellow Koreans, nor they with her. Weir's description of the setting illustrates the economic disparities within Minneapolis and also within the state's Asian American population. They performed in a lot full of broken glass and gravel near a housing project that was almost certainly the Riverside Plaza, a set of high-rise, low-income apartment buildings that, when I was a student at nearby Augsburg College in the 1990s, were referred to by locals with the deeply classist and racist monikers "Crack Stacks" and "Ghetto in the Sky." Weir and Lee would have been wearing happi coats, obi, and hachimaki, marking their performance as Japanese, but the woman nevertheless recognized them as Korean. Weir's description of the encounter as "heartbreaking" may signal a number of things: that she felt empathy for a woman she perceived as isolated, that she (and perhaps Heewon) wanted to communicate with her, and that it was meaningful to be recognized as Korean despite being ensconced in a performance with Japanese costumes and drumming. Kim Park Nelson ascribes the term "invisible Asians" to Korean American adoptees to signal that, as Koreans raised in white families, they often are not recognized as racial minorities by their families or as real Koreans by other Korean Americans. Thus, each of these scenarios in which Korean adoptee performers are recognized as Korean is significant.

Moreover, these scenarios involving Weir, Lee, the boy, and the elderly woman reveal another side of outreach performance. Though the potential exists for Orientalist scenarios to unfold, taiko outreach performances are also a site for recognition and connection between Asian Americans in a racial landscape that is often largely white. Beyond the ways these two anecdotes highlight the impact of being recognized as Korean within a Japanese or pan-Asian performance context, these two encounters also demonstrate the economic disparities between two subsets of Korean immigrants: adoptees, who enter the United States with the economic and cultural privileges of whiteness (though not, as recent cases have shown, of citizenship), and adult immigrants, some of whom enter the country without English language skills or the benefits and privileges of whiteness, regardless of class status.[75] These examples, then, highlight the heterogeneity within the Korean American and Asian American populations of Minnesota.

The history of Korean adoption in the United States can be seen as its own scenario of discovery in which Westerners play savior and discoverer to a foreign other. Transnational adoption of Korean children by (mostly white) American parents results from a tangle of military, missionary, and diplomatic relationships between the United States and Korea that started in the mid-twentieth century. Jae Ran Kim demonstrates how Protestant Christianity and racism were interwoven in transnational adoption pioneer Harry Holt's efforts to bring orphaned Korean children to the United States in the 1950s during the U.S. military occupation. In 1955 a trip to Korea inspired Holt, an Oregon businessman, to adopt not only the two orphans his family had been sponsoring monetarily but six more as well. A religious epiphany and the adoption of these eight children (which required hurdling federal immigration roadblocks) were the impetus to open the Holt Adoption Agency soon thereafter.[76] Undergirding transnational adoption was a white American desire to save Korean orphans. Kim writes, "The underlying theme of Protestant Christian philosophy in the welfare of children of color was often that of 'saving the heathen' from the 'dark or savage' ways of their native cultures." She cites a letter that Holt wrote saying, "We would ask all of you who are Christians to pray to God that he will give us the wisdom and strength and the power to deliver his little children from the cold and misery and darkness of Korea."[77] Thus, U.S. military occupation of Korea and the racism embedded in the Christian missionary attitude toward Korea as cold, miserable, and dark set the stage for the boom in adoption from Korea that was to follow.

Minnesota, in particular, boasted social conditions that allowed Korean adoption to flourish there. As Park Nelson notes, Minnesota's history of strong social welfare programs, combined with its racial homogeneity and relatively progressive racial politics throughout the early twentieth century, very likely created favorable conditions for the formation of adoption agencies that facilitated transnational and transracial adoptions. In particular, agencies such as the Children's Home Society and Lutheran Social Services, both of which began facilitating Korean adoptions in the 1950s and 1960s, began promoting Korean adoption over domestic adoption by the 1970s. "By the mid 1980s," Park Nelson writes, "so many Korean children were arriving in Minnesota" that Korean adoption no longer would isolate adoptive parents but rather "could actually connect them and their families with a growing community of adoptive families raising children from Korea."[78] Minnesota is now a hub for adoptee communities, support networks, organizations, and research. It is, therefore, not mere coincidence that Mu Daiko, as a group based in Minneapolis, has been home to a number of Korean adoptee taiko players. Rather, their presence reflects part of what makes Minnesota's Asian American community distinctive.

To explore more deeply how adoptees theorize their experiences as taiko players, I turn now to a close reading of a spoken-word piece written and performed by Mu Daiko member Su-Yoon Ko. When I interviewed Ko for the book, it was on her return to Minneapolis after eleven years abroad in Seoul, where she lived, worked, and co-founded Adoptee Solidarity Korea, an adoptee-led organization that advocated for the rights of adoptees in Korea. She had written and performed "Reaching," the poem I analyze here, at a time when she was performing frequently in schools as a taiko player with Mu Daiko, as an actor with Theater Mu, and as a Kabuki performer. The poem reflects her struggle with the reasons why she was spending so much time in schools when she had hated being a student. She told me, "Doing as many taiko outreaches as I did, I think I could've easily burned out, but 'Reaching' helped me explore and understand my feelings about the outreaches and the conflicting feelings that started to pop up about them." My analysis blends a textual reading with details that emerged from having seen her perform it live (albeit many years ago) and is aided by a video recording of the performance, a multimedia collaboration with photographer Charissa Uemura.[79]

Su-Yoon Ko stands in dim light with papers in her hand. She is alone on stage, but black-and-white images of taiko players engaged in multiple stages of the performance process occupy a large screen behind her. The photographs show taiko players mid-jump, smiling at audiences, folding their costumes, and moving drums and equipment through the cold Minnesota winters (see figure 3.6). Ko's words explore her ambivalence about being a Korean American adoptee performing taiko in Minnesota schools. Tonight is Asian theme night at the now-defunct monthly women-only cabaret Vulva Riot in Minneapolis. "Asian theme night" might sound as if it could go terribly wrong, but the evening's lineup has been thoughtfully curated by local Asian American artist and activist Juliana Pegues to include artists working in a variety of forms (including a few Mu Daiko numbers), several of whom deliver incisive cultural critique. Before a racially mixed audience, Ko recounts the struggles and joys of teaching elementary students the rhythms and Japanese vocabulary of taiko.

Lines spoken early in the piece reflect the narrator's boredom and frustration with taiko outreach. She says,

> As we roll the taiko into the third suburban gym that day
> the walls laced with loneliness
> I wonder what I'm doing there
> [. . .]
> banging drums to ancient rhythms
> dishing out the diversity for the day

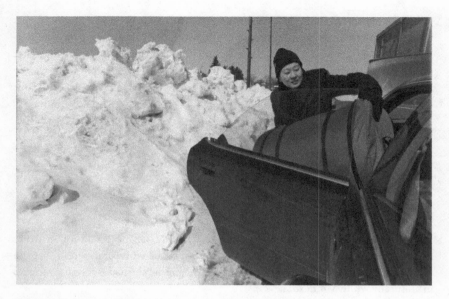

Figure 3.6. Su-Yoon Ko loading taiko equipment in a Minnesota winter. Photo by Charissa Uemura. Used with permission.

> and I sigh when I realize how tired I am of
> teaching white people Japanese translations
> feeding fuel to any philes fires. [80]

Ko's words evoke the monotony of outreach performance—often simple repertoire, sometimes repeated several times a day—and implicates herself in the potentially exoticizing scenarios that taiko sometimes entails. Further inscribing herself in the Orientalist spectacle of "kung fu-ish gear," which potentially refers to both taiko and Kabuki, she does not represent herself as being passively displayed, but instead writes herself into the poem as an agent of Orientalism, actively dishing, teaching, and feeding Asian stereotypes to her audiences, which, she indicates, may be or become Asiaphiles.

A motif of eyes and eye contact emerges in the next few stanzas as she describes her interactions with the Asian American students in her audiences. Eyes are a pervasive synecdoche for Asian racialization, "slanted" eyes standing in for a host of other phenotypic traits. Eyes also function as a pathway of identification, allowing people to communicate recognition and shame:

> I search out the yellow
> and try to make eye contact
> All too often they look away
> ashamed these Asians are acting so Asian

When Ko utters the words "so Asian," her lip curls in a sneer of disgust: she performs the alienation the children mentioned in the poem (and almost certainly she herself at their age) felt when they recognized other Asian Americans. In the lines that follow she identifies with this shame, detailing how, growing up in a white family in the Minneapolis suburbs, she too hoped *not* to be associated with other Asians, cherishing instead the "compliment" of being told she blends in. She continues,

> During Q and A there's the inevitable "What are you?"
> Once, after I say I'm a Korean Adoptee
> one little girl lights up and her whisper "I'm a Korean adoptee!"
> wraps around my heart like a gift
> and reminds me who I'm reaching to.

In answer to her earlier rumination about teaching Japanese culture to white Minnesotans, Ko realizes she needs to be in front of the white children so that she can also reach the Asian Americans, to be the role model she had lacked growing up in culturally white Minnesota.

The poem's evocation of eye contact, sometimes unmet, demonstrates the complexity of racial identification and Ko's uneven success in connecting with Asian American audiences in Minnesota. Eye contact as it is deployed here also highlights the agency of the outreach performer in returning the audience's stare, disrupting the assumption of an easy one-way Orientalist gaze in taiko performance. The piece further exposes the imperfect metaphor of outreach performance, that the performers deliver knowledge or enlightenment to listeners. Not only is Ko reaching to her audiences, but Ko herself is being reached, too. While Ko's delivery of the poem communicates both her disidentification with taiko's Orientalist potential and the pride she feels in reaching out to Asian American students, Uemura's photographs simultaneously demonstrate the multilayered processes of performing taiko.[81]

Early in the poem, Ko wonders why she dresses up in "kung fu–ish" gear to teach white students about Japan, whether through Kabuki or taiko. As the poem winds down, Ko (as narrator) gives herself the answer:

> I'm not there to educate the white ones,
> helping to sharpen their appropriation skills.
> I'm there for the yellow brown
> to be the role model I never had
> I want them to know
> they are more than a morning of show and tell
> more than Japan day
> Asian month
> I want to armor them with information
> I want them to be so full of love of self their eyes unfold from the burden[82]

She acknowledges the threat of appropriation and white audiences' Orientalist desire to consume Asian forms, but also concludes that she can decide for herself how she uses taiko. The events she lists—"show and tell," "Japan day," and "Asian month"—are familiar to taiko players as the kinds of events at which we are asked to perform. But here they also evoke the burden of representation that Asian Americans (and other minorities) are often asked to carry in mainstream white American contexts. Ko's poem layers such exoticism with her own agency—indeed, her desire to instill agency in her intended audience. And she returns to imagery of eyes, to give them a way to see their own worth, to release them from their burden of representation.

Commenting on her process in writing the piece, Ko said that she thinks of "Reaching" as a "love poem to Asians, to myself, to my younger self." She explained that when she was in school, because she was so lonely there, all she dreamed about was not being in school. This piece is in many ways a rumination on how she ended up spending so much time there as a performer. She says that performing with Mu helped her understand more about herself as an Asian American, and more specifically, as a Korean adoptee. These experiences of performing Asian America led her to move to Korea and eventually to advocate for other Korean adoptees living there.[83] The stakes of outreach performance, then, were high, both for her own life and for those in the audience. The "so what" of drumming is nothing less than empowering Asian Americans with information, with love, and with self-worth. Here, her visibility as both an Asian American woman and a Korean adoptee, coupled with knowledge of their own worth, arms her young Asian American spectators against the casual violence of everyday racism.

Su-Yoon Ko's "Reaching" and Jennifer Weir's recollections of encounters with Korean audience members elucidate both the challenges and the pleasures of performing Asian America in the Midwest. In particular, Ko's ambivalence about being a Korean adoptee performing an art form from Japan with an Asian American taiko group in Minnesota prompts questions about what it means to perform Asian America at the turn of the twenty-first century in the Midwest, which is historically and demographically distinct from the coasts. Minnesota has vibrant Asian American communities with thriving arts groups and advocacy organizations, but not on the same scale as those in California or New York. Isolation and recognition are surely not alien to Asian Americans in any location, but they recur as themes for Minnesotan taiko players.

These outreach scenarios also challenge notions of what it means to be Minnesotan. Weir's interactions with the Korean adoptee boy, as well as Ko's poetic theorizing of her experiences, highlight what may be a uniquely Minnesotan experience, given the demographic significance of Korean adoptees there. While Minnesota may seldom be imagined as anything but a state populated by white Scandinavians, Mu Daiko's outreach performances show otherwise: they challenge this image of the state. Performing in scenarios that unfold on- and offstage, Mu Daiko members embody a heterogeneous, yet distinctly Minnesotan Asian

America. Outreach audiences are never homogenous, and performers' affective responses serve as evidence that outreach performance is more than multicultural exchange; it gives performers, in Taylor's words, "room to maneuver."

The outreach scenarios I have described in this chapter reveal a range of attitudes on the part of audiences and performers, particularly as they center on race and ethnicity. Repertoires of racism and of recognition are enacted in words, gestures, and silences by performers and spectators. These performances are never for the first time and carry with them power and knowledge. While this chapter has focused primarily on Asian Americans performing in mostly white contexts, Chapter 4 examines white and black performers practicing a largely Asian American art form. As it widens its scope beyond Mu Daiko, it also focuses more tightly on women in its interrogation of the intersections between race and gender in taiko performance.

CHAPTER 4

Practicing Ambivalence

White and Black Women in Asian American Performance

In 2004 five members of San Francisco Taiko Dojo (SFTD) made an appearance on the short-lived ABC sitcom *Life with Bonnie*, in which comedian Bonnie Hunt plays Bonnie Molloy, whose attempts to balance her domestic life with her job as host of a Chicago morning talk show provide the show's dramatic thrust.[1] In the fictional world of this episode, Seiichi Tanaka (well known among taiko players as a founder of North American taiko) and four other dojo members perform on Molloy's show. When the episode was broadcast, it represented a rare moment in which taiko was featured on national television in the United States. It aired years before clips could be shared easily via social media; that many people in the taiko community had heard about it before it was broadcast attests to the rarity and excitement of that moment. A fellow Mu Daiko member recorded the episode directly from network television to a VHS tape and gave it to me to watch. At rehearsal, we were all excited to see the scene and proud that the little-known art form that we practiced would gain some national recognition. The clip, comic and straightforward, showcases the SFTD drummers as themselves, in contrast to the sinister and more overtly Orientalist depiction of the same group in the film *Rising Sun* about a decade earlier.[2]

In the episode, five men pound on large barrel drums while the camera cuts between shots of the drummers and Bonnie's appreciative gaze. The men drum together in synch, Tanaka playing the enormous o-daiko, a large drum suspended from a wooden frame, his back facing the audience while the other four play smaller drums and face the audience. When they have finished their performance, Bonnie walks over to chat with the performers and to take a quick taiko lesson. In her high heels she is a good six inches taller than Tanaka, and she slings one arm over his shoulders with avuncular familiarity. Bonnie's working-woman image, complete with a crisp tan coat, nylons, and smart glasses, contrasts starkly with Tanaka's traditional garb. Next to Bonnie's bright blondness and urban modernity, Tanaka is configured as decidedly, stereotypically Asian, wrapped from head to toe in sturdy, unstructured cotton. Though only two of the other four drummers are Asian American (one is Latino and one is white), their uniform masculinity and matching Japanese costumes cement a reading of the group as Asian.

As she sheds her coat for a quick taiko lesson, Bonnie jokes, "Let me get this off. I'm sweating just watching you—[turning to one of the young Asian American men] you, personally." The four younger men play a straight beat as Tanaka-sensei coaches her on how to play the o-daiko. She holds the large bachi at an unnatural angle, which makes her seem strangely weak. Her upright stance and high-heeled shoes render her unbalanced next to the wide martial arts stances the men adopt during their performance. When she dons the Japanese happi coat that Tanaka offers her, it serves only to heighten the contrast between her and the men: her bright yellow borrowed costume pops out against the dark blues and reds that the men wear. Her lack of rhythm and her contrasting colors, the eyeglasses that signify reason and intellect, serve to juxtapose rather than integrate her with the performers whose embodied-ness is on display. Moreover, the scene reworks the familiar trope of the seductive Asian woman caught up in the gaze of the white male viewer and his stand-in, the camera. In this case a white woman occupies the desiring position, and a group of younger male drummers, figured as racially other, are the objects of her gaze. After Tanaka plays a short, intense solo on the o-daiko, Bonnie remarks, "Next time, buy me dinner first, know what I mean?" Her sexual innuendo acknowledges the erotic facets of taiko and its performers. Still, Bonnie's attempts at cougar-like humor are as awkward as her drumming and ultimately reinforce her status as outsider.

The scene constructs a white woman's attempt to play taiko as awkward, comic, and more or less unnatural. Bonnie, the scene seems to suggest, is just too white to play taiko. Indeed, white women taiko players often do stand out in ways this scene exaggerates—when they perform taiko, particularly in groups with a majority of Asian Americans, their whiteness becomes visible and often remarkable. Richard Dyer, Peggy Phelan, and others have demonstrated the ways whiteness often goes "unmarked" or becomes normalized within mainstream U.S. culture.[3] But because taiko reads as Asian owing to its Japanese aesthetic and its preponderance of Asian American players, whiteness is often not invisible but remarkable on the taiko stage. One aim of this chapter is to address the cultural ambivalence produced by white women's involvement in North American taiko. I contend that in addition to the feminist and Orientalist pleasures it may afford them, taiko also offers opportunities for white performers' usually unmarked racialization to be unsettled in productive ways. The *Life with Bonnie* scene highlights both race and gender as axes along which white women negotiate taiko performance, but it does not account for their self-reflection on their practice or their responses to audience expectations of authenticity in this art form.

If whiteness becomes remarkable on the taiko stage, how and when does blackness appear or disappear? Although African Americans participate in U.S. taiko in very small numbers, focusing solely on the relation between white and Asian American taiko players would risk eclipsing the presence of other people of color. Among the most recognizable black American players is Art Lee, whose taiko career led him from California to Japan, where he now leads a group called Wadaiko Tokara.[4] The experiences of the very few black women playing in taiko groups in North America shed light on the ways in which Asian Americans and African Americans are triangulated along with white people in U.S. culture. In her foundational essay "The Racial Triangulation of Asian Americans," Claire Jean Kim argues that Asian Americans are constellated in a "field of racial positions" in relation to white and black people such that, while Asian Americans are "valorized" or considered superior to blacks (but inferior to whites), they are also more "civically ostracized" or seen as further outside American culture than are black people.[5] By centering both white and black women's negotiations of Asian American performance, this chapter explores a question that surfaces periodically within the taiko community: how do players who are not Asian American fit within taiko, an art form that is ostensibly open to everyone but also tied to Japanese tradition and Asian American communities? In particular, how do white and black women and their audiences co-constitute the gendered and racialized dimensions of Asian American performance?

In preceding chapters I have demonstrated how taiko is tied to activism and examined Asian American taiko players' negotiations of everyday racism and Orientalist performance contexts. I have also elucidated the improvisations and interventions that taiko groups and individual players make in a variety of scenarios, both on and off stage. In this chapter I explore the intersections of gender and race in taiko performance by turning to the experiences of white and black taiko players. Why focus on whiteness in a study of Asian American performance and cultural politics? The TCA's 2016 Taiko Census data suggest that 18 percent of taiko players in the United States are white women.[6] Black women, as noted above, participate at a lower rate. More important, perhaps, than quantifying the significance of these players' experiences is that this analysis comes at a time when broader national conversations about white privilege, white fragility, and white supremacy have come to the fore.[7] When Asian American performance studies scholarship turns to white performers, it is often within a context of yellowface performance and cross-racial casting issues in theatrical productions.[8] And whereas Dyer and others focus on whiteness in representation, this chapter contributes to scholarship on whiteness and performance by exploring the materiality and embodiment of white racialization as intersectional, lived experience in the practice and performance of taiko.

I argue throughout this book that taiko constitutes a crucial enactment of Asian American cultural politics, but this enactment is not performed by Asian Americans alone. Rather, a range of corporealities and ideologies co-constitute Asian America via the practice, performance, and consumption of taiko.[9] My experiences as a white woman taiko player deeply influence this chapter, which relies on interviews and autoethnography, because taiko has been and continues to be a crucial means by which I have come to understand race in the United States. In this chapter, I argue that this participation activates anxieties related to such issues as authenticity, belonging, and colorblindness, even as it expands gendered ways of moving through the world. In what follows, I contextualize this work within an ongoing conversation in the North American taiko community about race and belonging. I then turn to the intersections between race and gender through analyses of first white women's and then black women's experiences as taiko players. In the final section, I trace the history of Iris Shiraishi's song, "Torii," to demonstrate how alienation can be a productive step toward developing cross-racial intimacies.

"YOU'RE A TAIKO PLAYER?"

In North America, taiko performers are diverse in terms of race, ethnicity, gender, sexuality, and age. There are no practice-wide restrictions on who can participate, even if individual groups determine membership in a variety of ways. Many taiko groups include people from a variety of identity positions, yet taiko has clear roots in both Japanese culture and in Japanese American and Japanese Canadian communities. In particular, the participation of white performers throughout the United States and Canada has been the subject of discussion at regional and national taiko gatherings, between audiences and performers, and among players.[10]

The growing presence of non-Asian players has gained attention since early in the twenty-first century. In 2003 the North American Taiko Conference offered a series of discussion sessions dedicated to pressing issues in the taiko community. Among them was a well-attended session titled "YOU're a Taiko Player? Playing a Japanese Drum When You're Not Japanese." The blurb for the session reads:

> It is estimated that nearly half of all of the taiko performers [in North America] are not of Japanese heritage, and out of that, half of those are not of Asian descent at all. Taiko is seen, however, as still a very Japanese instrument and practice by many practitioners and also our audiences. Are there identity politics? Are there questions of cultural confusion? Do we even think about it, because we play simply for the love of taiko?[11]

That the session was part of the taiko community's largest regular gathering attests to its importance and indicates some concern about the way taiko evolves as an art form, who can claim ownership of it, and who can perform it legitimately. The blurb estimates that approximately one-fourth of taiko players were non-Asian in 2003. This figure, though it cannot be taken as authoritative, provides at least a sense that there was a significant number of taiko players at that time who did not identify as Asian American. From my observations at subsequent taiko conferences, it appears that the percentage has risen in the years since. The presence of this workshop highlights anxiety about this demographic trend, namely, that taiko will become disconnected in the popular imagination from its roots in racial struggle and Asian American identity formation.

Nonetheless, the North American Taiko Conference boasts a visible Asian American presence. While it cannot encompass all taiko players' experiences, the biennial conference is one of the best touchstones available for understanding who is involved in taiko in the United States and Canada. It was at NATC that the white female taiko player Nicole Stansbury, a member of Odaiko Sonora in Tucson, Arizona, really understood taiko as a Japanese American art form. When I asked, in an interview, if there is any part of her experience with taiko that makes her feel like part of an Asian American community, she replied, "At Conference. . . . But really not in Tucson that much because there's—it's very different coming to conference where you realize that it's—yes, it is a Japanese American art form originally, and you're like, 'Oh Yeah!' "[12] Odaiko Sonora is an ensemble founded in 2002 by two women, Karen Falkenstrom and Rome Hamner. Its membership is multiethnic, but it does not describe itself as an Asian American taiko group. Although the members are very involved in local community activities, including the elaborate, annual All Soul's Day celebration, they are not as specifically linked to Asian American communities as San Jose Taiko or Mu Daiko. Stansbury's realization at NATC that taiko is an Asian American or Japanese American art form suggests not only that the gathering reflects high Asian American participation in taiko but also that the racial breakdown of the taiko community as a whole is not necessarily reflected in all local groups.

It is safe to say that at the North American Taiko Conference, Asian Americans are present in larger numbers than many people from the middle of the country are accustomed to. Moreover, as part of the opening ceremony at each conference, one of the board members shares a slide show and lecture about the history of taiko in North America. For returning participants the history is well-known, but the information is new to first-time conference-goers who often comprise about half of the participants. The history reflected in the slides is unmistakably a story of Asian Americans discovering and developing a new Japanese American diasporic tradition at the same time as the relatively new "Asian American" identity emerged in the United States. For Stansbury, taiko's Asian Americanness does not mean she does not belong. Although the conference made her aware of taiko's Japanese American roots, with time she came to feel welcome as a white woman. She says, "One of my first conferences I felt just a little off that I'm this little white chick coming to perform at Taiko Ten [Community Concert]. But I was never *made* to feel that way. So it was, in general it's been a very welcoming thing." The trepidation she felt did not come from how others behaved toward her but from her own new awareness of being in the minority. Her rhetorical move of referring to herself as a little white chick signals her awareness that her whiteness makes her stand out, yet the diminutive terms "little" and "white" also minimize the importance of her whiteness, or perhaps belie some anxiety about being in the minority or talking about race.

For some, taiko has always been not simply an Asian American but a specifically Japanese American activity. The session description for "YOU're a Taiko Player?" had framed taiko as "very much a Japanese instrument." The discussion touched on a range of experiences and perspectives: I heard one twenty-something Japanese American panelist indicate that for her, taiko was one of her Japanese activities, and she was somewhat baffled that white people would want to do it at all. Having grown up on the West Coast, where there are large Japanese American communities, she saw taiko as a "JA thing," much like Japanese language lessons, something she did with her Japanese American friends. Another panelist explained that playing taiko in a group that was largely Asian American gave him, a white man, the welcome if uncomfortable experience of being in the minority.

Others in the room approached taiko differently. A middle-aged white woman complained that she was excluded from performing desirable parts in her group because she was not Japanese. Of the many people in the room, some of the most vocal were a few white performers who felt they were being treated unfairly. I was surprised that the conversation had taken this turn toward what Robin DiAngelo might call white fragility, "a state in which even a minimum amount of racial stress becomes intolerable, triggering a range of defensive moves."[13] In contrast to the white man who acknowledged his own racial otherness within his group, which apparently was mostly Asian American, the women in question betrayed no awareness of their white privilege, nor did they make any attempt to reconcile their experiences with other kinds of exclusion. Much of the session was devoted to their issues, despite the range of people and perspectives in the room.

White fragility is not simply a personal or individual state of being. DiAngelo argues that it is a cultural phenomenon undergirded by systemic factors in American society, including a culture of racial segregation, widespread discourses of universalism and individualism that tacitly favor white perspectives, and a host of other attitudes that aid white people's sense of entitlement. That white people are largely unaware of how these advantages operate in their lives gives rise to defensive behaviors.[14] Mu Daiko member Rachel Gorton attended the session with me, and afterward we discussed the issues that arose, including the ways our experiences differed from those of the players who had complained. In an email, she later wrote, "I'm wondering if part of this was that we were firmly rooted in the history of taiko from the beginning and throughout the years, we both shared the history and cultural aspects of taiko hundreds of times at outreaches." That is, as members of a group with a strong Asian American affiliation, we benefited from the group's inclusion of white performers but also from the knowledge that the group circulated about the roots of taiko. Further, she noted (and I agree) that she and I, as white women, had assumed that "we [were] guests in this art form."[15] Within this discussion about taiko and identity, as with such discussions within North American taiko at large, these apparently competing perspectives on taiko (as Japanese American, Asian American, universal, and so on) reveal racial tensions.

The presence of white performers in taiko is a point of discussion not only among taiko players, but also between audiences and players. When I performed with Mu Daiko, there were some years when I was one of only two or three white performers onstage and others when the group was nearly evenly split between white and Asian American players. In a card Rachel Gorton gave me for the opening night of an annual Mu Daiko concert she wrote, "Break a leg to my matching bookend!" Her comment reflected something of an inside joke. Having begun to play taiko at around the same time, we had comparable skill levels and physicality, and we were often paired together in pieces that called for some sort of visual symmetry. In the context of Mu Daiko, Rachel and I were noticeably white, with our blond hair and Scandinavian looks. We are of a roughly similar age, height, and complexion. We do not *really* look alike: our faces, hairstyles, and bodies are actually quite different. We would not ordinarily be mistaken for one another, yet as performers with Mu Daiko, audience members have gotten us confused. For example, an audience member once asked me about my children (I don't have any, but Rachel does), and sometimes when new taiko students attended our classes, they mistakenly believed they saw one of us perform when it was actually the other. I am not suggesting that all white women look alike in taiko; in other words, this is not a reversal of the stereotype that all Asians look alike. Rather, I want to emphasize that there is just enough similarity between Rachel and me that audiences read us as similar and that race—specifically, our whiteness—is one way in which audiences made sense of us in performance.

The presence of white performers in Mu Daiko further reveals audience expectations and responses to race onstage. I give two brief examples. During my early years with Mu Daiko, I performed with two Japanese American women in a small building at the Minnesota State Fair. As we packed up our drums afterward, an older white man approached me and joked, "I've never seen a blond Japanese woman before!" His comment recalled Richard Dyer's assertion that blond hair and blue eyes are considered "uniquely white, to the degree that a non-white person with such features is considered, usually literally, to be remarkable."[16] But this man did not, of course, mistake me for an actual blond Japanese woman. Blondness functions as a synecdoche for whiteness, hair color standing in for a range of phenotypic markers of race, and his comment simply implied that I didn't make sense; I stood out as a white person in what he read as a Japanese context. It would be the first of many comments I fielded from other white people, statements or questions made in a joking but conspiratorial tone. A common reading of these encounters would be that people are simply trying to be friendly and to relate to the people they have seen onstage. It is true that spectators who comment on my whiteness never do so with hostility; in fact, most of the time, they treat it as a kind of inside joke. Yet the matter-of-factness of the scenario is exactly the point. We both know the script; there is an assumed understanding between us as white people that there are certain spaces in which we don't belong. The audience member's comment even functions as a subtle reminder that I—to paraphrase John Garvey and Noel Ignatiev—have violated the terms of membership in the white race by acting Japanese.[17] Such comments also imply that my presence has interrupted the audience's expectation of seeing Asian bodies, or perhaps it has betrayed Mu Daiko's simple Minnesotanness, for all its Japanese posturing.

The second example further reveals how whiteness interrupts audience expectations. For several years, Mu Daiko performed each December at the Southern Theatre in Minneapolis and afterward we formed a reception line in the lobby to greet the audience. One Friday night, a white woman approached Rachel and me, shook each of our hands warmly, and said, "I was so disappointed to see you blond girls up there, but then you were both so *good!*" The warmth of her tone contrasted disconcertingly with her message. This woman probably expected to see only Asian faces in a Japanese drumming concert, and our presence disrupted her expectation of authenticity. Her use of the word "blond" rather than the more precise term "white" is again significant: although she felt comfortable talking to us about how she apprehended our bodies onstage, she did not directly name the racial dimensions of her observations. Rather, she spoke in a code that, on the surface, seems more polite; commenting on hair color is more socially acceptable than speaking directly about race. In the moment, we thanked her (after all, she had implied that our performance skills had redeemed our inappropriate racial performance). As we hashed over the incident in the dressing room later, it became clear that no one else had received such a comment, including the two white men who had also performed that night.

Such offstage scenarios between performer and audience suggest that white performers disrupt audiences' expectations of authenticity (read: Asian bodies) in taiko performance. And, of course, the racial aspect of the comments is rarely about whiteness; rather, it is about Asianness. As dance scholar Rosemary Candelario writes, a performance must seem exotic and distant in order to provide Orientalist pleasure, and anything that makes the performance familiar, such as white bodies, interrupts the fantasy.[18] This woman's disappointment implies an expectation of Orientalist pleasure that our bodies did not immediately provide, regardless of our skills.

Questions of race and belonging, then, arise both within the taiko community and among spectators. The conversation that developed at the "YOU're a Taiko Player?" discussion at NATC shows that there are multiple and overlapping ways for players to approach their practice of taiko. For some, it is firmly ensconced in a range of activities associated with Japanese American life, while for others it is an opportunity to examine one's own white privilege. Yet as the complaints of the two white women reveal, taiko also operates within a culture that values universalism, which typically benefits white people. Moreover, spectators bring their ideas of belonging when they see a taiko performance, and sometimes the presence of white performers unsettles spectators' expectations of Asian authenticity. But there is a gendered dimension to some of these comments as well, since women's bodies are always available for comment and evaluation in ways that men's bodies seldom are.

In the following section I turn my focus to white women's words to explore the intersections between whiteness and womanhood as material, lived experience.

TAIKO, MOBILITY, AND WHITE WOMANHOOD

This section considers the intersections among gender, race, and social mobility in white women's experiences in taiko.[19] Not unlike white women in the nineteenth and early twentieth centuries who looked to Asian styles and forms to enable new kinds of femininity, contemporary white women see taiko as allowing for a range of femininities to be embodied and performed.[20] Much like the Asian American women in Mu Daiko for whom outreach performances produced ambivalence (see Chapter 3), white women also experience cultural ambivalence because of their triangulated position as both possessing white privilege and living as women under patriarchy.[21]

White women's access to taiko depends on their social mobility, whereas the pleasure they take in it has much to do with how the form lets them move *as* women. Whiteness, according to Richard Dyer, is tied narratively and visually to "order, rationality, [and] rigidity," even death, and this emphasis on reason and the brain contrasts with "black disorder, irrationality and looseness."[22] (Recall, for example, Bonnie Hunt's rigid, upright posture and kinesthetic awkwardness as she attempted to play the giant taiko in front of her.) Feminist theater scholar Kate Davy extends Dyer's formulation of whiteness to account more fully for gender, positing that Dyer's theorization of whiteness as a "disembodied or beyond-the-body state of abstractness . . . is not entirely available to white women, since femininity itself is characterized by embodiedness."[23] She writes, "The white woman's privilege . . . can be understood in terms of her mobility." That is, she can move along a continuum ranging from embodiedness (associated with people of color) to rationality (associated with white men), though she can never fully occupy the "unembodied dimension of white masculinity, for 'to embody' is still her definition and destiny."[24] While Davy asserts that white women move representationally between whiteness and blackness (neither she nor Dyer accounts for racialization outside this binary), I consider white women's social and kinesthetic mobility, as well.

As compared to black women, white and Asian American women may have more similarities than differences in terms of social mobility. Asian American racialization in the late twentieth and early twenty-first centuries often positions Asian Americans in proximity to whiteness owing to economic success and to "their purported overrepresentation in such fields as Western classical music, engineering, science, and technology."[25] In common parlance, Asian Americans can at times claim status as "honorary whites." Moreover, whiteness, in Dyer's formulation, is signaled by rigidity in the U.S. context; Asians are often depicted as excessively rigid, even robotic. Much as Asian American women have done, white women taiko players often articulate their enjoyment of taiko as stemming, at least in part, from a gendered sense of embodiment.[26] Despite the similarities that both groups may have in terms of social mobility, the social pressures on white, black, and Asian American women are different.

My own trajectory, as well as Rachel Gorton's, hinged on both class and social mobility related to whiteness. Like many other taiko performers and students, we had the leisure time to attend and money to pay for ongoing classes. After becoming performing members, although we no longer paid class fees, we were able to dedicate several hours per day, often up to five days per week, to rehearsing or teaching. Each of us is college-educated, comes from a middle-class background, and had developed, via various routes, an interest in Asian and Asian American cultures.[27] Having come of age in the 1990s, we were and are part of a culture that valued a celebratory multiculturalism.

My introduction to taiko hinged on privileges associated with middle-class status. I began playing taiko because, just after college, I was working as a stage manager with Theater Mu, which had recently started the taiko group Mu Daiko. In December 1998 I stage-managed the group's concert; in January 1999 I took my first taiko class. But before I worked with Theater Mu, I had been introduced to taiko while an intern at the Children's Theater Company in Minneapolis, a position I secured in order to fulfill the requirements of the theater program at Augsburg College. Even my involvement with Theater Mu happened thanks to a recommendation from my faculty advisor, a founding member of the company who was married to its first artistic director, Rick Shiomi. I list all these details to highlight that my access to taiko was completely dependent on being college-educated, having access to social and employment networks, and having the social mobility associated with middle-class whiteness to experiment with new artistic interests.

Rachel Gorton's route to taiko, though different from mine, was no less dependent on middle-class social mobility. She, too, began playing taiko in January 1999, after seeing the same concert that prompted me to play. She had grown up in the suburbs of Minneapolis and attended St. Olaf College in Northfield, Minnesota. She and her husband (who was also a member of Mu Daiko for several years) had just returned from a three-year stint living in Japan as teachers for the Japan Exchange and Teaching Programme (JET), a project supported by Japan's Ministry of Education.[28] The Gortons lived in Toyama prefecture, where they taught English in a high school and took up the martial art *aikido* in their spare time. On returning to Minnesota they attended the December 1998 Mu Daiko concert with a friend from the JET program. Gorton told me that for her and her husband, playing taiko became an important way of maintaining a connection with Japan. But that was not the only reason for the pleasure that Rachel took in taiko. She also mentioned that, particularly in her first year of performing with Mu Daiko, the intensity of learning new repertoire and of maintaining an intensive rehearsal schedule re-created some of the rhythms of her life in Japan. She enjoyed feeling like "everything was kind of out of control and really difficult."[29] Within a few years Rachel started to build drums in her garage, along with her husband, Drew, and other Mu Daiko members and taiko enthusiasts.

My engagement with taiko hinged not on its Japanese roots specifically but, rather, on what I perceived as its clean-lined Asian aesthetics and its feminist and queer social possibilities. These are, of course, desires I can only fully articulate in the present and are only a few of the many reasons why I began to play. When I first saw Mu Daiko perform I had no plans to become a member, not because I held any sophisticated beliefs about white privilege and cultural appropriation but simply because I did not know if this was something white people *did*. A four-week class would be a fun thing to say I had done, but I never expected to be considered as a performing member. When I began taking classes, Mu Daiko's performing group was comprised entirely of Asian American members, and given its affiliation with an Asian American theater company, it seemed reasonable to me that they might keep it that way. Initially I was drawn to the power of the performers, both for the clean lines of their unison drumming and for seeing the women in particular burst into furious action during solos. As I have written elsewhere, the aesthetics of taiko also appealed to my feminist, bisexual, lesbian self, who liked the ways in which it drew attention to women's physicality without overly feminizing or exoticizing their bodies.[30] As I began to learn more about taiko by playing, talking to other players, and eventually attending conferences, other aspects of it appealed to me. I enjoyed the sense of ritual and discipline that is often part of taiko practice, if not always part of Mu Daiko's practices. As I mentioned in the preface, some of my attraction to taiko was part of an unarticulated Orientalism; I saw the etiquette and hierarchies of taiko practice as non-Western, different from the kinds of discipline taught in athletics and theater.[31] It was only through working closely with Asian American theater and taiko artists—and later, taking Asian American studies courses in graduate school—that I developed a more sophisticated way of thinking about my participation. But my sense of racial alienation—in the Brechtian sense of having an awareness of the material circumstances of my participation—was present from the beginning, even if not fully articulated.

Rachel Gorton, despite having lived in Japan and being familiar with some of the Japanese vocabulary and etiquette used in taiko, described her awareness of her whiteness as a source of anxiety. In terms of how taiko affected her everyday life and the way others viewed her, playing taiko imbued her with a feeling of being interesting and of doing "something different." It allowed her to exceed the boundaries of a "typical Scandinavian" woman who grew up in Minnesota. Having recently left the group at the time of our interview in 2009, she said that without taiko she felt "just kind of boring."[32] Although these reasons for playing were only a few among many others, taiko did offer something of an antidote to the perceived banality of white suburban life. In her ethnographic study of white women's attitudes toward their racial identity, Ruth Frankenberg noted that her subjects' "descriptions of the contents of white culture were thin, to say the least." Participants made comparisons between white culture and items such as bread and mayonnaise and used terms such as "blah" and "bland" to "signify paleness or neutrality." To Frankenberg, these descriptions pointed to the "lack of vitality . . . and [to the] homogeneity" of white culture.[33] Here whiteness is experienced not as rigidity or death (as in Dyer's formulation) but as a kind of lack, an absence of interest.

When I interviewed Rachel, she recalled nearly verbatim the comment that an audience member had made about being disappointed by our whiteness. We had both made light of that encounter at the time, but it had clearly resonated with both of us. In my case, I was motivated to write about it. Rachel said, "I always felt personally ... like I had to work harder and I had to kind of overcome [being white] ... like it was a detriment in a way." In Chapter 3 I established that Mu Daiko outreach performances often carry the expectation that the group will deliver Japanese or Asian American culture to its audiences. About these performances in particular, Rachel noted, "I always felt, like personally for me, like I had to sell it a little bit more because I wasn't Japanese. . . . I wasn't even Asian American, and so therefore there was that element of 'look at that funny blonde woman.'" She laughed as she continued, "Like, you know, she doesn't belong there." In the context of Mu Daiko, and specifically public performances in which taiko carries an expectation of Japanese or Asian American authenticity, Rachel noticed and felt whiteness not as abstract but as material, lived experience. She also thought that perhaps her previous training in aikido had prepared her well for learning taiko and that her good technique could keep audience members from noticing that she was "shockingly blonde" in contrast to the others.[34] Far from being unmarked in this context, she experienced her whiteness as remarkable, that is, as something she expected audiences to recognize and remark upon, whether or not they did in any given circumstance.

Whiteness was not the only thing that made Rachel feel like an outsider in Mu Daiko. She described to me the difficulties she faced in her early years with the group when she was pregnant with and caring for her first child. Playing taiko gave her a feeling of "invincibility" that she carried into other aspects of her life, and being part of an art form that embraces powerful women was a "constant source of pride" for her.[35] She made her comment about invincibility while relating that taiko—along with competing in triathlons—helped her manage issues with body image that she, like many women, has experienced. Taiko allowed her to "transcend" feelings of insecurity about her body and mobilize it to "actually . . . look powerful and graceful."

Although she cited taiko as empowering to her as a woman, it is also clear that her involvement in taiko was not free of the pressures that women face in the workplace, education, and other sectors when they start families. She reminded me, for example, that she played in Mu Daiko's December concert (the second one for both of us) after giving birth to her son in late September and then undergoing a painful medical procedure. She said she "didn't want to get left behind" in terms of the group's development, and she continued to rehearse, perform, attend the taiko conference, and build drums, all while pregnant and then caring for a newborn. She described this period as one in which she endured both physical pain and a great deal of stress trying to balance work, family, and leisure. And because others in the group at that time were not raising small children, she felt, in her words, "quite different" from other players. So although her gender identity per se did not make her an outsider in a group at least half of whose members were women, her experience of feeling like an outsider was nonetheless distinctly gendered.

The struggles that Rachel outlined in our 2009 interview were echoed by other women in 2015 in a discussion session called "Women and Empowerment" at the North American Taiko Conference in Las Vegas, at a panel discussion titled "Women and Taiko" at Mu Daiko's Minnesota Taiko Festival in 2017, and again at the "Women and Taiko" Summer Taiko Institute in San Diego in August 2017. Among the many topics covered in these discussions, the gendered nature of how women and men navigate their lives differently as taiko players and in general became a strong theme. Participants listed child-rearing labor, societally enforced behavior patterns, and casual sexism among issues that women taiko players deal with, often unacknowledged, in their groups. The specifics vary from player to player, but it is clear that Rachel's experience is not an isolated one and that taiko is not immune to widespread structural sexism.

In addition, however, white women experience taiko as a practice that allows them greater mobility and freedom. For Nicole Stansbury of Odaiko Sonora and Jodaiko, taiko has less rigidly defined gender roles than do other movement practices she'd been involved in. Before she joined the Arizona-based Odaiko Sonora, Stansbury performed with the modern dance troupe OTO Dance. In fact, her first contact with the taiko group in Tucson was through a collaborative performance between Odaiko Sonora and OTO Dance. Because of an injury she had sustained while doing aerial dance work, the creators of the taiko-dance collaboration asked Stansbury to learn some taiko rhythms rather than dance, and after that her involvement deepened to the point where now she is a full-time taiko player and teacher.

Before I interviewed Nicole at the 2015 North American Taiko Conference, I had met her twice: once when I and three other Mu Daiko women performed as guests in an Odaiko Sonora concert, the same one Nicole mentioned as her debut, and again when I traveled to Tucson on a research trip in 2009. Odaiko Sonora's founders had managed to build a successful company—and a set of their own drums—in a few short years. Our invitation to play was articulated as part of their effort to connect with other powerful women taiko players.[36]

For Stansbury, playing taiko allowed a more expansive range of gender performance than modern dance had allowed. She told me:

> I was a very strong, masculine dancer anyway so I was always told, "You dance like a man. You jump like a man." So coming into taiko was really actually good for me because I got to be grounded and strong, and that's fine, as opposed to "Come on. You need to work on being a little more feminine." Yeah. Not so much. So. It was nice to . . . no longer be told I was—and not like it ever bothered me. I loved being aggressive and fiery in my dancing. It's just [that] choreographers didn't always like me being aggressive and fiery.

Far from Bonnie Hunt's awkward attempts at drumming, Stansbury describes taiko as a good kinesthetic fit for her body and temperament. She is petite and athletic, with sandy brown pixie-cut hair, freckles, and an outgoing personality. Though it would be a stretch to call her masculine or butch, she has a tomboyish quality that toggles between sprightliness and intense groundedness. The wide-legged stances often used in taiko, the strength and volume associated more typically with masculinity, are what drew Stansbury to the form. Modern dance, too, draws on grounded physicality and deep emotion, but in Stansbury's experience, despite her rather petite size, she was always encouraged to be "a little more feminine" as a modern dancer. The physicality required of taiko matched her gendered sense of herself.

At the same time taiko satisfies her desire to perform gender in a way that feels natural, Stansbury's earlier description of herself as a "little white chick" at the North American Taiko Conference signals discomfort, if temporary, as a white woman practicing taiko. These simultaneous experiences of taiko's appeal to alternative versions of femininity and white women's outsider status coexist as ambivalence. For different women, these overlapping performances of race and gender materialize in different ways as audience expectations and societal pressures also exert themselves on performers.

For white women, the broad physicality and powerful sonic qualities of taiko allow for a wide range of gendered movements, even as it prompts them to experience and embody their racialization in new ways. Their participation is undergirded by a relatively wide field of social mobility that is afforded white women, even when they perceive racial barriers. Moreover, the presence of white performers on the taiko stage often disrupts audience expectations of authenticity (or authentically Asian bodies). Whereas for white women, playing taiko demands that they think about their white racialization, often for the first time, for the black women I interviewed, taiko is a space in which racism is downplayed in comparison to everyday life.

RACIAL TRIANGULATION TAIKO AND BLACK WOMEN

Amanda, a member of Soten Taiko in Des Moines, Iowa, wrote in an email to me, "It's hard to think of my personal experience playing taiko as remarkable in any way, except for the fact I get to play it at all in Des Moines, Iowa."[37] In the years since I began playing taiko in the late 1990s, opportunities to see and participate in the form in the Midwest have increased, though it remains more accessible in larger cities such as Minneapolis, Chicago, and St. Louis than in smaller ones. What makes Amanda's experience notable is that she is one of a small number of taiko players in North America who identify as black or African American. According to the 2016 Taiko Census, such performers (including mixed-race persons) made up less than 2 percent of respondents.[38] It is likely there are black players who did not complete the survey, but it is clear that participation by black taiko players in the United States and Canada remains comparatively low. The three women

I interviewed who identify, at least in part, as black perform in different parts of the country: one in California, one in Iowa, and one in Michigan. All three are mothers, all began playing as adults, and like the other participants I interviewed, all are college-educated. Some of the experiences these three women related to me overlap with those of white women, while others highlight the different processes of racialization for black women in the United States.

The relatively small number of black taiko players in North America obscures the musical and political connections between taiko, Asian American activism, and black political movements.[39] Many taiko groups cite American jazz and rock, both of which have roots in black musical styles, as musical influences. Perhaps most notably, Kenny Endo combines taiko music with his extensive expertise as a jazz musician and cites black jazz performers Gil Scott Heron, John Coltrane, and Miles Davis as early influences.[40] The Los Angeles–based Taikoproject, founded by Bryan Yamami, emerged as a group that infused its music and choreography with the aesthetics of hip-hop, a form rooted in black music and dance. But beyond the musical ties, sansei taiko players in the 1960s and 1970s describe the ways in which growing up in or near black neighborhoods in California formed their political consciousness. In her study of what she terms "pre-Movement" Japanese American radicals, Diane Fujino posits that the proximity of Japanese Americans to black communities was an important factor in setting the stage for such well-known Japanese American radical activists as Yuri Kochiyama, Mo Nishida, and Richard Aoki, who would become leaders of the Asian American movement.[41] This proximity, Fujino points out, "was not so much due to feelings of solidarity, but rather the result of structural and residential restrictions." Although many housing regulations (both official and unofficial) steered buyers into racially segregated areas, it was after Japanese Americans returned to cities such as Los Angeles and San Francisco after internment that they found themselves living in or near African American neighborhoods.[42] Similar narratives emerge in Life History Interviews conducted by JANM for the 2005 exhibit *Big Drum: Taiko in the US*. Russell Baba, who performed with SFTD and later founded Shasta Taiko, Roy Hirabayashi of San Jose Taiko, and George Abe of Kinnara Taiko all made connections between black political movements and their own politicization at about the time they adopted taiko as an Asian American practice.[43]

These histories are not necessarily ones that resonate with the three black women I interviewed, all of whom are younger than the pioneers of North American taiko. In my observations, with few exceptions, the political and aesthetic connections between taiko and black expressive culture are not ones that most taiko players acknowledge widely.[44] Rather, the black women I interviewed were drawn not to political or activist aspects of taiko but to its empowering physicality and to the specifically Japanese aspects of the art form. In other words, they seem to be drawn to similar aspects of taiko that interest white performers, including its Orientalist appeal.

Sascha Molina performs, teaches, and serves as Assistant Director for Sacramento Taiko Dan in California. When we spoke, she was candid about how unique her experiences as a black woman in taiko are. I met Sascha face-to-face for the first time on the day of our interview at the 2015 North American Taiko Conference in Las Vegas. Sascha grew up in a middle-class black family in California. She does not prefer the term "African American" because she "know[s] nothing of Africa," but rather describes herself as black and "multicultural," having grown up in a Mexican neighborhood with a racially diverse school environment that included mostly Mexican, Filipino, and white classmates. She said, "I guess I identify as black but I don't."[45] She explained that though her parents are black, her family does not come from the American South or observe traditions often associated with southern black heritage. Her husband is mixed-race (Mexican-Indian and Norwegian) but doesn't identify as Mexican, and their son is mixed-race. As she elaborated in the interview, others often have expectations of her when they see a black woman playing taiko that do not align with her embodied experience.

Molina tied her taiko practice to a long-standing interest in Japanese culture that stemmed from a having Japanese American friend in high school and later having decided to learn the Japanese language. She was drawn to what she described as "cultural traditions" of Japan. That is, she seems to enjoy learning about Japanese culture as much as she enjoys practicing taiko. And in particular, she says, "It's the traditional things that move me. . . . The other stuff, sure it's cool, but I get real moved by the traditional stuff."[46] In this context, her reference to "traditional" music hews to many North American taiko players' use of the word to describe the kinds of regional Japanese festival music and drumming traditions that pre-date the twentieth-century phenomenon of *kumi-daiko*, or ensemble drumming. Sascha's teacher at Sacramento Taiko Dan, Tiffany Tamaribuchi, studies and teaches some of these traditional styles of Japanese drum music in addition to playing North American kumi-daiko (see figure 4.1). Much as Rachel described taiko as supplementing her life as a white woman in the Midwest, Sascha understands taiko as part of Japanese culture, which she sees as distinctly different and more interesting than the cultural aspects of her own upbringing.

Sascha began playing with Sacramento Taiko Dan in 2007 after an Internet search led her to the group. By taking classes and learning from DVDs, she quickly worked her way up to teaching and performing. She assists Tamaribuchi, the group's founder, with teaching classes and giving public workshops and was also part of the organizing team for the Women and Taiko summer intensive in 2017. Sascha initially felt that her performance options would be limited because she was not Asian or Asian American. She mentioned that in "one particular instance, someone said, 'Oh, you can't do that. You can't tour with this group because they won't take you because you're black. You have to be Asian.'" Later, she said, the group in question (which she did not name) hired a black woman performer, and Sascha made a decision not to listen to what others said but rather to simply proceed with her training, saying "You have to follow your heart whether some people understand or some people don't." Whether the unnamed group she mentioned took race into consideration is not really the point. Sascha had already assumed that there was a racial barrier to her progress in taiko, even before another person had reinforced the belief. She thus

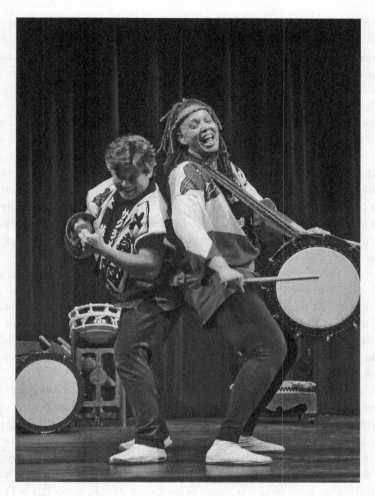

Figure 4.1. Sascha Molina, right, performs with her teacher, Tiffany Tamaribuchi, left, in a Sacramento Taiko Dan concert. Photo by Katharine Saunders. Used with permission.

experienced her blackness as a form of alienation from taiko and perceived herself as having limited professional mobility as a taiko player before forging ahead with her plans. This is not to suggest that the barriers were in her imagination, but to point to her experience of alienation resulting from racial difference.

Sascha's blackness is a source of curiosity for audience members, who often ask questions or articulate their assumptions as to why she plays taiko. When I asked about instances when race and ethnicity emerged in relation to her participation in taiko, she told me,

> I'm definitely noticeable and memorable because I am so odd. It's like, "She's tall, her hair, she's so different. Like, who is she and how did she get—why?" So, people

actually mostly assume that I'm married to a Japanese person. And my son's very ambiguous, so many people think that he's part Japanese, when he's not at all. So, yeah, I think . . . they want to try to understand. And so they just start making stuff up. But, yeah, [being asked why I play taiko is] a big question that I get often at these shows.

Sascha referred to her race, her height, and her hair as sources of oddness on stage. In addition to being a black woman among, presumably, Asian American and white performers, Sascha is quite tall and wears her hair in braids, a hairstyle that signals blackness. Figure 4.1 shows that Sascha is at least a head taller than her teacher, Tiffany Tamaribuchi, and her hairstyle differs from the usual ponytails or short hair worn by other women taiko players. She theorized that spectators' curiosity and assumptions about her interest in taiko are simply their attempts to understand what they are seeing. As with audience members who question white women's participation in taiko, jokingly or not, Molina's encounters are based on audience's expectations that they will see only Asian bodies in a taiko performance. Like some of the Mu Daiko members interviewed in Chapter 3, Sascha did not necessarily see encounters with audiences as rooted in racism. Rather, she said, "I *am* interesting. It is like, 'Why are you playing taiko?' Like, I don't mind those questions at all. I really don't." Yet it is clear that audiences have trouble making sense of black bodies on the taiko stage—and want to ascribe to them some connection to Japaneseness in order to do so.

When audience members question her about playing taiko, they map their assumptions onto her by announcing their expectations of black bodies in motion. She related that being an outsider in taiko echoes her experience of playing sports when she was younger. Referring to her participation in volleyball and swimming, sports not typically associated with black athletes, she described people's response: "It's 'Oh, you don't play basketball?' "[47] Similarly, in reference to taiko, she says, "[P]eople have asked me this: 'Well, why not African dance?' [she laughs] Like, African Dance? Why would I do that? I'm not interested in that. But—or African drums, actually. I get that a lot. 'Why not African drums?' There's no big sticks!" Thus when audiences articulate their surprise at seeing her on the taiko stage, they not only reveal their expectations of Asian authenticity. They also articulate their expectations of what black bodies in motion should be doing instead. Her experiences thus coincide with white women's in terms of feeling or being told they don't belong, but they also demonstrate the limits of colorblindness when spectators go a step further to articulate their assumptions about where black bodies belong.

Shereen Youngblood had also participated in athletics and music in high school and college before she started playing taiko. She was born in Detroit, where she lives and performs with Godaiko Drummers, a community group associated with the Great Lakes Taiko Center (GLTC), based in the Detroit suburb of Northville (known locally as Novi). She identifies as bi-racial, with a father who is black and mother who is Native American. Shereen's reasons for playing taiko, like Sascha's, were connected to an interest in Japanese culture. Her daughter, who was five at the time, was enrolled in a language immersion school and was learning Japanese. In an effort to reinforce language acquisition, she sought out Japanese activities for her daughter. When she saw the GLTC group perform at a Japan Festival at a local high school, she thought taiko might be a good activity for both herself and her daughter.[48] The GLTC, which offers classes and supports two performing groups, the professional-level Raion Taiko and the community group Godaiko Drummers is not framed as Asian American but as Japanese. That is, founders Brian and Mayumi Sole learned taiko in Japan, where Mayumi was born, and their annual concerts are emceed in both Japanese and English. Thus, for Shereen to assume that taiko could reinforce her daughter's Japanese language acquisition was perhaps more accurate in the context of GLTC than it would be with other North American taiko groups.

Gender informs Shereen's continued participation in taiko on multiple levels. Besides engaging in the activity with her daughter, seeing Hono-O-Daiko, a dynamic and virtuosic all-women's group from Japan, perform, inspired her to continue. The group has served as mentors to the Soles and GLTC, and, Shereen said, "When I saw those women specifically . . . it really just inspired me even more to say, you know, try and see . . . how far you can go." Shereen noted that although the form is male-dominated (which is true in Japan if not in the United States), in Godaiko Drummers, "it's nothing but women the majority of the time." Moreover, "By having taiko as what I would call a hobby, it has really pulled me away from always doing work. And that was one of the things that I was always constantly doing was work." As a social worker in child welfare, her work could easily overwhelm her life, and taiko gives her an outlet from this demanding job.

When I asked Shereen if playing taiko ever highlights issues of race, she replied, "I haven't experienced any type of negativity because of race or gender." She added, however, that she does not want to reinforce any of the myriad negative stereotypes of African Americans in the media. She said, "I've had so many positive black role models that it just kind of always befuddles me to think how negatively we're portrayed. But for me, that wasn't my world. That was not what I saw or experienced." For the most part, when she is singled out by audience members, it is because they assume that she is the English speaker among Japanese speakers. Somewhat as I have been singled out as a white woman when performing with Mu Daiko, Shereen's blackness signals "American" to audiences who assume that the group's Asian members do not speak English. In the case of Godaiko, there are, indeed, members whose primary language is Japanese, because the group draws on Northville's relatively large population of Japanese nationals. Nonetheless, a black performer's being seen as either a linguistic or cultural translator for Asian members triangulates African Americans as more culturally "inside" U.S. culture than are Asian Americans.[49]

Amanda of Soten Daiko, whose surname is withheld, similarly acknowledges racism as a problem, but sees taiko as relatively immune to it. Her group, whose name means "Blue Sky Taiko," was founded in 2011 in Des Moines, Iowa. She had been introduced to taiko as a college student in Minnesota, and then saw the Japanese ensemble Kodo perform. She said "I'm from a small rural town in Kansas, which I left as soon as I could. I played the piano and violin, but wasn't allowed to play the drums because my mother thought it wasn't lady-like." She added, "I know that there is a stereotype of who plays Taiko, a young buff Japanese man, but Taiko is for those it speaks to." With regard to how playing taiko has highlighted issues of race, Amanda's answer had some similarities with Shereen's. She said,

> This is a difficult question to answer. Race is something that other people inflict on us. On a normal day I don't think about the fact that I am a woman of color unless I'm somewhere where I feel like I stick out, or I'm reading the news. The US has a huge race problem that seems to be getting worse, so I do think about it more currently than I did a few years ago.

But, she told me, "[W]hen it comes to Taiko, I don't feel any negativity from anyone regarding my race. I come from a mixed Black/White/Native American background, but none of the Taiko players I've met seem to care." She noted that sometimes when none of the Japanese performers are present, audience members ask whether the group has Japanese players, but she did not mention any other racial encounters. Shereen and Amanda don't feel that doing taiko marks them as exceptional or remarkable; rather, it is a space in which they are comparatively free from the kinds of anti-black racism they encounter in the media.[50] Both also stated that they get asked to speak for their Asian American co-performers or asked about the absence of Japanese performers, indicating that their blackness signals Americanness in the context of taiko performance.

Taken as a whole, these interviews shore up a number of insights about taiko as an embodied practice that produces ambivalence about race and gender. It is clear that, far from operating in a colorblind context, taiko highlights issues of race, in particular, allowing whiteness to become legible in performance—but also demonstrating how blackness signals Americanness, in accordance with Claire Jean Kim's theory that though Asian Americans may be seen as superior to black Americans in some ways, they are seen as further outside American culture. Further, while many women see taiko as a feminist practice that allows for a positive self-image and a range of possible gender performances, women's experiences within taiko groups are gendered in ways that reflect structural sexism present in the wider culture.

MOVING TOGETHER: "TORII" AND PRODUCTIVE ALIENATION

North American taiko offers a great deal of potential for cross-racial encounter through rehearsal processes, performance experiences, and interactions with audiences. Even the Bonnie Hunt clip that opened the chapter dramatizes a moment of intimacy between a white woman and, primarily, a Japanese American man as he teaches her a new skill. While many white women taiko players engage deeply with the form, taking classes, performing, and attending conferences, it is nonetheless possible to be a dedicated taiko player without ever learning much about the form's history in North America or engaging with its Asian Americanist genealogies. American Studies scholar Sunaina Maira critiques such context-less involvement in her study of white American women's uneven investments in belly dance practice and performance, arguing that the dance's liberatory and (mostly white) feminist possibilities obscure the imperialist and liberal multiculturalist structures that encourage a cultural, but not a political, engagement with Arab or Middle Eastern cultures, a practice she names "Orientalist feminism."[51] In a similar vein, Yutian Wong maintains that the recent surge of interest in Asian forms such as yoga, tai chi, and belly dance—as consumerized practices and as supposed alternatives to Western tastes, behaviors, and beliefs—render invisible the Asian and Asian American bodies that also practice, teach, and produce such forms and whose histories and labor made them widely available for consumption in the first place.[52] Taiko potentially appeals to its practitioners on several of these levels—as culture, spirituality, athleticism, and artistic practice—yet it in many contexts, it is still tied to Asian American communities and practitioners.

In the final pages of this chapter, I explore how white women might engage with taiko as a site of cross-racial intimacy and move beyond the apolitical form of Orientalist feminism described by Maira. How and when might performing Asian America be a conscious act of anti-racism rather than a form of cultural amnesia? The moments of ambivalence, awkwardness, and outsider-ness that arise in taiko become opportunities to make this deeper engagement. Brechtian alienation, on which I elaborate below, is a productive position on the basis of which to nurture critical observation rather than either the unmitigated pleasure of Orientalist embodiment or the denial that comes with seeing taiko as universal. While the instances in which whiteness becomes visible and noteworthy onstage may highlight audience expectations and performers' own moments of alienation, the dynamics of the rehearsal space are also informed by race, as well as gender and sexuality. I turn to the ways race and gender informed the composition and learning process of the song "Torii," Iris Shiraishi's first composition for taiko.

Rachel Gorton and I learned "Torii" soon after we joined Mu Daiko. Shiraishi wrote it for herself and another Asian American woman, Jennifer Weir. The representational meanings are not my focus, but rather how the process of learning and embodying the piece asks performers to engage its Asian Americanist impulses and, perhaps, to recognize and reckon with their own identities in the process.

In order to describe the phenomenon of a performer negotiating her own identity in relation to a performance piece and its social and historical context, I draw loosely on German playwright and theorist Bertolt Brecht's concept of alienation. Rather than ask actors to fully identify with the characters they play, as was the prevailing realist approach to acting when he wrote in the 1930s, Brecht wanted actors to use an intellectual and critical approach to their characters, with an awareness that the choices they make should communicate information not only about the character's psyche but about the "entire structure of society at a particular (transient) time."[53] When taiko players perform, they do not inhabit a character or interpret a play script, but they can quickly essentialize what taiko is and what Japan is—or, in essence, slip into an Orientalist mindset in which one easily and uncritically adopts practices simply because they are, or seem, Japanese. Alternatively, taiko players (or for that matter, anyone learning a new art form) can choose to approach it critically and to understand that their performance is a historical and political one. That is, their participation resonates with the entire structure of society. Only by adopting a critical stance about an art form can we remain aware of its history, in this case the relation of taiko to its cultural politics and our relation to the form's history. Like dance scholar Anthea Kraut, I believe that "it should be all of our responsibilities to learn and transmit the histories of the forms and formations we inherit and perpetuate."[54]

I shake my limbs nervously as I wait in the stage left wings. I can see Rachel across the stage waiting on the other side. It is our first time performing "Torii" in public. Three drums sit center stage, the largest one upstage center, the apex of a triangle formed with two other drums downstage, an inverted V opening out to the audience. The drums sit *betta*-style, meaning that one drumhead rests on the floor, while the other faces straight to the ceiling. Watching each other closely, Rachel and I walk toward each other to center stage and take our places on opposite sides of the upstage center drum. We make eye contact, and in unison we sink into a wide-legged stance and unfold our arms in a downward-sloping angle. A beat later, we raise both arms at an angle above our heads, the tips of our bachi almost meeting above and between us. We hold them there only momentarily before we begin to play the slow, soft first beats of the song.

"Torii" was written to honor the memory of Esther Torii Suzuki, a Japanese American woman known for her lifelong commitment to Asian American and women's issues in the Twin Cities. When I learned to play "Torii," Iris Shiraishi had been a member of Mu Daiko since 1997. Born in Hawai'i, Shiraishi came to the mainland for graduate school in Iowa and later moved to St. Paul, Minnesota, with her husband. A musician and composer by training, Shiraishi had not written music for ten years and was nervous about composing for taiko after having studied the form for only three years. She had been "reluctant to even think about composing" for taiko until her friend and colleague Suzuki passed away in 1999. Besides referring to Suzuki's middle name, "Torii" is also the Japanese word that describes gates found at the entrances to Shinto shrines and sometimes Buddhist temples. As Shiraishi often explains when she introduces the song to audiences, Suzuki had always encouraged people to challenge themselves, and Shiraishi wrote this piece to push herself to a new level of performing.[55]

I remember seeing Shiraishi and Jennifer Weir perform a workshop version of "Torii" when it was in development before it received its premiere in Mu Daiko's

2000 annual concert. The power and ferocity that these two Asian American women channeled for this song amazed me. As they continued to perform it over the years and their onstage connection grew, the song became more and more powerful. After executing the ritual formality of the opening phrases, the women play several bars of rhythms that are soft and easy hits to the drumhead and rim. The straight base beat then continues while each takes her turn playing variations on one shared drum. The pace and volume increase, and eventually, each woman flies through a series of spins, arms out to the side, propelling her back and forth between the center drum and the one on her side of the stage (see figures 4.2a through 4.2c). Then they are facing each other across the shared drum again, this time with a faster pace, stronger hits, and a sparkle in their eyes. As they pick up the pace, they play new variations on the initial theme, their arms pounding noticeably harder on the drums. They fly again between drums, arms pinwheeling around their bodies, voices filling short silences with ferocious yells. While one moves, the other beats the drum loudly, yelling "Yeahhhhhh!" Finally the drummers' tempo winds down to slower, but still powerful, hits to the drum, until the two face each other again on the big drum and play the same five slow beats with which they had begun, ending the song with upstage arm raised at a forty-five degree angle and eyes lifted to follow it.

Although it would not be obvious from simply watching a performance, the development of "Torii" is inextricable from Asian American arts and activism in the Twin Cities. The song's namesake had inspired Shiraishi in the short time they knew each other. Suzuki's family had been interned at a camp in Portland, Oregon, during World War II, and she was able to leave the camp to become the first Japanese American student to attend Macalester College in St. Paul, Minnesota, where the Lealtad-Suzuki Center now stands.[56] As Shiraishi recalled, Suzuki was involved in a number of activist organizations, including several dedicated to Asian American women's issues. The two met when they took part in an educational outreach performance with Theater Mu called the "Mu View," a program that included a mix of storytelling and taiko drumming. Suzuki was one of the storytellers, sharing stories from her life, and Shiraishi was one of the drummers. "She really kind of took me under her wing . . . I'm so not political a person," Shiraishi said, but Suzuki had a way of drawing people into organizations and other events, including two protests calling attention to the Orientalist plot and racist casting of Miss Saigon when it played at Twin Cities venues. Suzuki's death was somewhat unexpected. "It was heartbreaking because even though I didn't know her really well, she was the one that really grabbed me and put me into this . . . Asian American community," Shiraishi told me. Writing "Torii" was her way to say a "meaningful goodbye" and to memorialize the influence that Suzuki had on her and the area's Asian American community. She included elements in the song that, at the time, were very challenging for her such as big arm movements, fast spins, and sticking that required her to lead with her left hand. When she was creating the piece, Shiraishi said, "it was always, like, with this feeling like [Esther] would look down and say, 'Okay, that's good. You're doing something to challenge yourself.' That was a benediction."[57]

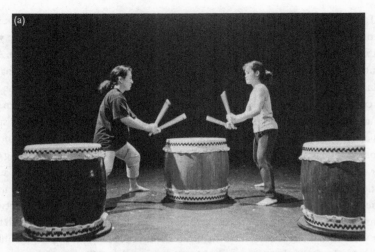

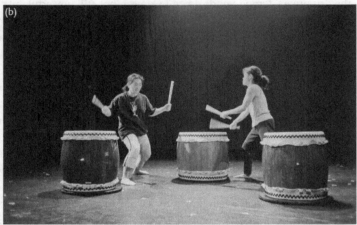

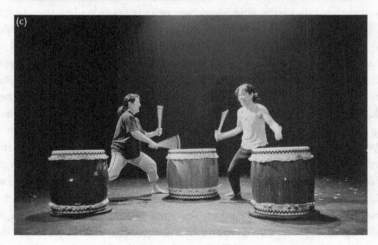

Figures 4.2a–c. Jennifer Weir (left) and Iris Shiraishi (right) rehearse "Torii" in Minneapolis. Photos by Charissa Uemura. Used with permission.

In addition to its roots in Asian American activism, the song's history also highlights the bonds between women. Not only was it written by one woman to honor the memory of another, but for several years, only women performed it. "Torii" is at once an intimate duet that relies on a rhythmic and emotional connection between the two performers and one that showcases the power and strength of the players. The wide, sweeping arm movements that propel the players from one drum to the other make these two relatively small women seem larger than life. Sections of the song that include hard, hammer-like hits to the center of the drum highlight the strength it takes to play. Whenever she composes songs, Shiraishi noted, she often finds it difficult to see them performed by players other than those who originated their parts or roles, particularly when she has little personal connection to the new performers.

When Rachel and I learned "Torii," we did so without the expectation that we would perform it. Simply because we liked the song, we began to stay after Mu Daiko rehearsals and learned it by watching a shaky VHS tape on a tiny television in the company's rehearsal space. We fast-forwarded and rewound sections of the tape countless times, learning the sticking, the spins, and the *kiai*, the vocalizations that are part of the song. Once we had the foundations down, we would occasionally stay after regular rehearsal to play it together, at first along with the recording on the tiny screen, and later on our own. When we eventually performed it, we were nervous because we associated it so closely with Jen and Iris's version.

We played it at a student recital (a lower-stakes situation than the more formal annual concert). It felt like a big deal, a rite of passage. It was a favorite among group members, and it was difficult for our playing level. The two performers rely on each other for a consistent rhythm and for energy and support, their rhythms interlock in a non-obvious way, and their movements are precisely timed. The photos in figures 4.3a and 4.3b capture the sense of speed and movement that

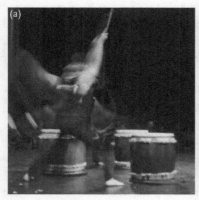
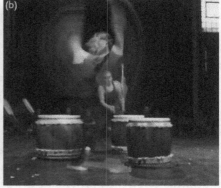

Figures 4.3a–b. Angela Ahlgren and Rachel Gorton perform "Torii" at a Mu Daiko student recital, Minneapolis. Photo by Drew Gorton. Used with permission.

the song requires. Rachel recalled that she had always been in her comfort zone keeping a steady beat in the background and staying out of the limelight. With "Torii," she said, "my discomfort came with only two of us carrying it all. There was no hiding, no escape, no interlude. The minute we walked on stage it was full throttle. . . . And I think that's what made it so powerful."[58] But the "big deal" of being able to perform it was about more than our mere ability to do so; it was also clear that the song was important to Iris. Playing the song for an audience, hearing Iris introduce it and talk to the audience about Suzuki—her friend and also a beloved member of the Twin Cities Asian American community, which comprised much of our audience—reminded us that playing the song carried a sense of responsibility: to the composer, to the song's namesake, and to those in the audience who remembered Suzuki and her activism.

Playing the song at that time was immensely pleasurable, even empowering, not only because it engendered the sense of accomplishment and mastery that comes from learning something technically difficult but also because the song demands power and ferocity—and demands them of women performers. At the same time, understanding the song's connections to Asian American activism, even if those connections are indirect, invites (but of course does not require) performers to critically examine their own role in the composition. As women, Gorton and I fit within Shiraishi's vision of showcasing women's power. When I interviewed Shiraishi, she noted that many of her songs can be seen as explorations of women's power onstage. "Torii" was the first song in which Mu Daiko intentionally placed women center stage, but later, she wrote other songs that featured women, both in roles that evoked power and those that emphasized softness and grace, qualities more often associated with femininity. She said, "I've always personally loved that Mu Daiko has been a predominately female group. I've also loved that females, regardless of identification and orientation, are attracted to this kind of art-making and have ostensibly felt comfortable and fully integrated enough to stay and develop their talents in taiko."[59] For Shiraishi, the gender dynamics of Mu Daiko and taiko in general are integral to the pleasure it holds for her—it has both personal and political implications. In addition, her phrase "regardless of identification and orientation" signals that her definition of "woman" is inclusive, but not colorblind. Her practice of and vision for taiko, then, are informed by gender writ large and by women's power, which presumably includes white, as well as queer, women.

On the other hand, two Asian American women originally performed the piece, which was inspired by another Asian American woman whose activism motivated Shiraishi to compose for taiko. When two white women perform the piece, its representational politics shift, certainly, but it is also an opportunity to examine the ambivalence, the simultaneous empowerment and alienation, that emerges for the performers. To echo Nicole Stansbury's awareness of herself as a "little white chick" at the taiko conference, performing this particular song as a white woman at the very least opens up the possibility of alienation and thus of thinking through how I approach this song.

But part of harnessing alienation requires having or being willing to attain some knowledge about the work and its context. Iris told me that, in terms of group dynamics, knowledge of Asian American history and an understanding of otherness can be helpful. She wrote,

> When you and Rachel were in the group, I simply did not have a struggle with those issues of racial/ethnic balance. Maybe it was because I knew from first-hand experience, that you and Rachel knew about [Asian American] history, and more importantly, had first-hand experience about being the "other." Rachel through her Japan experience and you through your GLBTQ identification and also through your academic work [in Asian American studies].[60]

Here, she acknowledged the important role of experience and learning in producing what, for her, makes a successful taiko group. In addition to knowledge, she pointed out, people with experiences that are themselves potentially alienating such as being gay and living in a foreign country may provide some basic tools for understanding and even adopting an Asian Americanist approach to taiko. Experiences of queerness, outsider status, and racial otherness are not exactly parallel, but for Shiraishi they signal a person's willingness to understand difference and power, and to have undertaken significant self-reflection at one time or another.

Creating productive spaces that foster cross-racial intimacy, then, requires knowledge, experience, and a willingness to recognize and harness moments of alienation. To return briefly to the "YOU're a Taiko Player?" session, moments of exclusion that the women discussed can be more than an opportunity for complaint. A tradition that has grown quickly and in many directions in a short time, taiko provokes myriad questions about belonging, authenticity, race, gender, and more. Rather than proceed from a position of universalism that benefits white performers in their access to an array of performance cultures, white taiko players might instead harness such moments to ask questions about the form in which they are engaged, to understand its histories and the racial formations it engages, and foremost, to recognize the political importance in supporting Asian Americans in setting the terms for the taiko groups and performances they create.

WHAT NEXT?

To ignore the Orientalist impulses in the practice of taiko would be to ignore the fact that many spiritual, aesthetic, and performance trends based on Asian forms find popularity at the same time that Asian people in the United States are reviled both on the level of national rhetoric and in everyday attitudes. In the context of the taiko community, it often feels impolitic to point out the potentially Orientalist underpinnings of white women's involvement.[61] When I have presented material from this chapter at conferences, some listeners have told me that I am reading too much into things, that it's perfectly fine for white women to play taiko, and that I shouldn't worry so much about it. I disagree. I am not concerned about whether white women should be allowed to play taiko. Rather, I think it is important for all taiko players to reflect on their participation in the art form, to understand taiko's activist genealogies, and to apprehend their role in co-constituting Asian America via their involvement in (often expressed as love for) taiko. Thus, this reading of white women's and black women's participation diverges from the colorblind multiculturalist view that race shouldn't matter. Thinking through cultural ambivalence in taiko, then, is an unruly maneuver that seeks to connect North American taiko practitioners to broader conversations about appropriation, belonging, as well as whiteness and blackness.[62]

If taiko is an art form in which white women and black women stand out as remarkable, albeit in different ways, how might such an awareness shape our approach to taiko and to other aspects of our lives? In a follow-up email in 2017, Rachel explained that in the eight or so years she has been out of taiko, she has cultivated a willingness to "name, explore, and accept that [white privilege] is part of my life" and that she considers her work on education and technology as a "lever or catalyst to larger social change."[63] She connects the work she does now, speaking to and supporting educators, to her earlier work in taiko, including the experience of wrestling with white privilege. In a similar way, the experience of understanding not only my own whiteness but becoming familiar with the experiences of fellow taiko players who are people of color, shaped the paths I have taken in my scholarship and teaching. How taiko circulates in performers' lives and in audiences' desires informs the next chapter. Chapter 5 turns to the intersections of race, gender, and sexuality in taiko performance in examining how the women's group Jodaiko queers North American taiko.

CHAPTER 5

Butch Bodies, Big Drums

Queering North American Taiko

The sound of drumming rumbles from the stage as the five women of Jodaiko move and sweat with each other on the outdoor stage of Vancouver's 2009 Powell Street Festival. Since 2006 Jodaiko has been a mainstay of the long-running Japanese Canadian community festival's performance lineup, a major venue for taiko since the late 1970s. During the same weekend as the Powell Street Festival is the Queer Arts festival, a series of performances and art exhibits by and for LGBTQ community members.[1] Its several weeks' worth of programming coincides with Vancouver's LGBT Pride festival, which itself overlaps precisely with the dates of the Powell Street Festival. Since 2007 Jodaiko has been performing at both festivals. This chapter takes these overlapping festivals as a site for performing queer Asian America through taiko. Tiffany Tamaribuchi, the group's leader, is a high-profile taiko player with an international reputation as a performer and teacher, and Jodaiko is one of several groups with which she performs (see figure 5.1). It is also one of the few all-women's North American taiko groups and one of perhaps two or three groups consisting mainly of queer Asian American and Canadian women. This chapter explores how Jodaiko queers North American taiko and argues for sexuality as a key lens through which to approach taiko performance.

When the women of Jodaiko (roughly, "woman taiko" in Japanese) take the stage, they perform a mix of their own compositions and "traditional" taiko music, following the conventions of many taiko groups.[2] Much of the group's repertoire showcases the strength and power of the drummers. Their costumes reflect a North American taiko custom of performing in tapered indigo pants, matching aprons, and colorful happi coats (informal coats fastened with an obi, or sash). In these ways Jodaiko is a typical taiko group, but it is unique in other ways. In contrast to more established groups such as San Jose Taiko, Mu Daiko and another of Tamaribuchi's groups, Sacramento Taiko

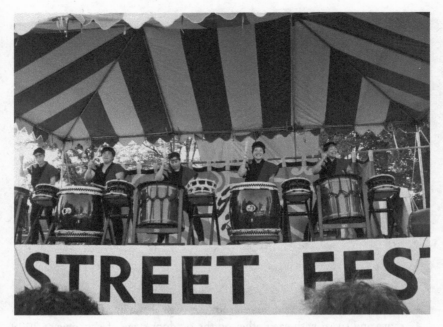

Figure 5.1. Left to right: Eileen Kage, Leslie Komori, Tiffany Tamaribuchi, Toyomi Yoshida, and Kristy Oshiro perform "Kokorozashi" at the 2009 Powell Street Festival. Photo by the author.

Dan, which have 501(c)(3) status, staff members, and a fairly regular membership, Jodaiko operates without the financial resources to compensate performers or sometimes even to cover travel expenses. Unlike many groups that are based in one city and rehearse together regularly all year round, Jodaiko functions as more of a pick-up group. Its geographically dispersed members seldom rehearse together except in the days leading up to a performance, when they spend time rehearsing and socializing intensively. While the pick-up arrangement is not in itself unique within taiko or music cultures more broadly, Jodaiko's provisional and temporary nature lends itself to a type of queer intimacy by bringing women together across national and ethnic borders in a community that is fluid (membership shifts as people's schedules permit), fleeting (just one week per year), and yet ongoing.[3]

Jodaiko is one of only a few all-women's groups in an art form in which women comprise 64 percent of participants. When I conducted fieldwork with Jodaiko between 2006 and 2009, it was the only group I was aware of made up entirely of queer-identified women. More recently, other groups and classes focused on or organized around sexuality have emerged, including the Genki Spark in Boston, RAW (Raging Asian Women) in Toronto, and Kristy Oshiro's taiko classes in the Sacramento area.[4] While Tamaribuchi does not call Jodaiko a queer or lesbian group, it performs in LGBTQ spaces and can be viewed through a queer lens. Addressing sexuality as a key facet of taiko performance highlights the erotic power of the form, as well as the gender and racial dynamics wrapped up in this performance practice.

This chapter draws on queer and feminist theories to highlight sexuality as a crucial component of taiko performance and spectatorship through three readings. First, I situate Jodaiko's emergence within the genealogy of North American taiko and argue that its formation responded to the seldom-acknowledged sexism among North American taiko groups. Second, through a reading of a group number, "Kokorozashi," at the Powell Street Festival, I posit that Jodaiko creates visibility for often-invisible queer Asian American women by their performance of butch uniformity, or what I call "homo-geneity." Finally, my close reading of group leader Tiffany Tamaribuchi's solo number "O-daiko" at the Pride in Art festival demonstrates how taiko performance can be queered through specific performance choices, context, and the complex and pleasurable relation between performer and spectator.

Like other performance practices, taiko calls attention to the drummer's body not only as an object to be consumed but also as a fiercely drumming body in motion. It points to the enduring issue, as dance scholar Yutian Wong writes, of "the multifaceted relationship between the body that dances with agency and the body seen dancing."[5] Ethnomusicologist and taiko player Deborah Wong writes that taiko can be a "passionately appealing" practice for Asian American women in its reconfiguration of "women's work," even as taiko performances remain open to Orientalist spectatorship.[6] Paul Yoon's work on taiko and Asian American masculinity in performance acknowledges the possibility for gay male spectatorship in certain taiko performances, but lesbian spectatorship and female masculinity in taiko have yet to be explored.[7] This chapter extends these analyses and draws on queer theory to argue that taiko can be viewed and practiced queerly.

Further, my focus on Jodaiko addresses the dearth of scholarship about women at the intersection of queer studies and dance and performance studies. In the introduction to her edited volume *Dancing Desires: Choreographing Sexualities On and Off the Stage*, Jane Desmond devotes a subheading to the question "Where are the women?"[8] More than a decade later, dance and performance scholarship concerning queer women, especially queer women of color, still lags behind that about (mostly white) gay men. Clare Croft's 2017 edited volume *Queer Dance: Meanings and Makings* begins to address this issue by making feminist and anti-racist projects central to the essays in the book and to the performances posted to the companion Web site. As Croft notes, "the pairing of white privilege and Euro-American centrism limits the range of dance forms categorized as queer, focusing on modern and ballet as though those are the only norms to queer."[9] In this chapter, my focus on queer spectatorship of this taiko group from a lesbian perspective, moreover, moves women of color and white women from the periphery to the center of queer performance as both performers and spectators. As before, rather than regard spectators and performers as occupying adjacent spheres, I show that spectators, too, participate in the scenarios that make up the larger context of the performance event, queer spectatorship, and Asian America.[10]

Seeing taiko queerly relies on both what is onstage and how the spectator is willing to engage with what she sees.[11] Scholarship about queer dance suggests that sexuality can become legible onstage via movement quality and spatial relationships, even in the absence of an explicitly queer narrative. Jane Desmond writes, "How one moves, and how one moves in relation to others, constitutes a public enactment of sexuality and gender."[12] Thomas DeFrantz notes that typical ways to read "queer" in dance include pointing to "excessive strength by women who lift men; flamboyant costuming or fantasy; men without women for entire movements of ballets; women without men for entire dances."[13] Both Desmond and DeFrantz indicate that one way spectators can read queerness onstage is in one dancing body's relation to another. I suggest that sometimes when one moves in relation to another, that other body might be the spectator's. In Stacy Wolf's parlance, the "lesbian spectator" does not necessarily have to be a lesbian but must simply be willing to view performance from a queer perspective.[14]

To a certain extent, I aim to discuss Orientalist and queer spectatorial practices together, as mutually constitutive elements of experiencing taiko performance. Deborah Wong and Paul Yoon have written about the potential for white American audiences to impose an Orientalist reading onto taiko performance.[15] But Wong also suggests that although "non-Asian spectators shift easily into the orientalist gaze," the "strength, control, [and] loudness" of taiko work to empower the Asian American, especially the Asian American woman, spectator.[16] I follow Wong's lead in "locating an erotics of taiko" that imagines alternative spectatorial positions by analyzing a kinesthetic spectatorship that disrupts the one-way, objectifying gaze.[17] If a queer spectator need not identify as queer, then perhaps white spectators with the willingness and knowledge to do so can also shift from an Orientalist gaze while watching Asian American performance. Although I theorize queer spectatorship from my own position as white and queer, I also suggest that Jodaiko's performances hold the possibility for the circulation of queer desire between the performers and audience members from a range of identity positions.

Jodaiko uses both original and traditional Japanese performance material, the latter of which is typically used to display the power of men's bodies, to reconfigure them in ways that can be read as queer performance. This chapter explores the queer pleasures of taiko for performers and spectators in order to ask how bodily performances of gender, race, and queerness circulate within taiko. To insist on the possibility of queer spectatorship in taiko performance is also to declare the existence of queer desires that circulate both onstage and among audience members. Queering North American taiko, then, is not only about the semiotics of the bodies onstage but also about the bodies of those who watch, listen, and participate in the performance. I argue that through performers' everyday performances of gender, performance choices, and the kinesthetic effects of taiko, Jodaiko's performances create visibility for queer Asian women and create possibilities for queer spectatorship of taiko.[18]

Jodaiko's visibility as an all-women's and de facto queer taiko group brings attention to issues of sexism and homophobia, which are present within taiko communities even if they are seldom discussed openly. Further, that it consists mainly of Asian players underscores a desire on the part of the performers to form community based on shared racial identification. As I have shown, many women taiko players experience the form as empowering and liberating. Professional taiko in Japan has been comparatively slow to fully incorporate women as drummers, as demonstrated by Chieko Kojima's experience with Kodo, but North American taiko has been inclusive of women since its early years. Nonetheless, gender-based inequities persist within taiko groups and in the larger networks that comprise the taiko community. Jodaiko was formed as a response to such inequities, in an attempt to create more opportunities for women to play.

Tiffany Tamaribuchi began her taiko training with the San Francisco Taiko Dojo in the late 1980s. Although many believe that women have always been involved in North American taiko, SFTD began as an all-male group made up of Japanese immigrants who gathered on a casual basis.[19] According to Mark Tusler, when two women began playing with the group in 1970, two years after SFTD was formed, Seiichi Tanaka had to "come to terms with his understanding of taiko performance as an all-male activity." He had initially operated under the assumption that women would not play drums, but he seemed to recognize that women's roles were changing in society at large.[20] That these two women performed publicly with the group in the early 1970s made a significant impression on women who saw them play. Jeanne Mercer, who joined SFTD in 1972, remembers seeing women playing taiko the first time she saw the ensemble at the San Francisco Cherry Blossom Festival. (She remembers the year as 1968 or 1969, but more likely it was 1970 or later if Tusler's data are correct.) Because this was the first time Mercer had seen taiko, seeing women on stage did not surprise her: "I mean, I thought that was just a great thing because why not? You know, why couldn't a woman be playing taiko?"[21] Unlike Tanaka, Mercer had never assumed that women could not play drums. From early in its history, then, women practiced and performed with Tanaka's group, but as many SFTD players have pointed out, inclusion did not necessarily translate to equal treatment.[22]

Although some of the women training with SFTD, a group whose style is often characterized by stereotypically masculine strength and aggression, were apparently strong players, they were not routinely chosen to play the more coveted roles.[23] For example, SFTD's signature song, "Tsunami," features soloists taking turns playing on the o-daiko, a very large drum that is the focal point for this number. It is hung sideways on a tall stand center stage, with two players, profiles to the audience, each playing on a head of the drum. Initially, two drummers play a slow opening section with set rhythms. Next, the remaining drummers take turns playing improvised solos on either side of the drum. With each new solo, the speed, intensity, and virtuosity build, with the flashiest and most powerful drummers ending the song. As Tamaribuchi recalled in an interview, women typically played the opening sequences, but rarely were they featured at the climax: "The hot stuff guys would come on at the end," she said.[24] The "hot stuff guys" are usually not only those who play faster and stronger but those whose performances highlight their stamina and strength through bared muscles, facial expressions, sinking low to the ground with effort, and in some cases using acrobatics to embellish their drumming. In this instance, the aesthetic of the song favors a performance of strength typically encouraged in male players, while the women are relegated to more somber, less physically demanding parts. To a large extent, this emphasis on strength and power has influenced Tamaribuchi's performance choices—she is now well known for playing the o-daiko, the type of drum and style of drumming used in "Tsunami." Yet at the time, she and other women were excluded from participating in the performances on an equal basis with the male performers.[25]

It was this dynamic of second-class participation that inspired Tamaribuchi and some of the other women from SFTD to begin playing together outside the dojo. This impetus coincided with invitations to perform at woman-centered events in the 1980s. In 1987 Tamaribuchi had only recently begun training with SFTD, commuting between her home in Sacramento and the dojo in San Francisco on a regular basis. As a student at California State University at Sacramento, she was approached about performing at a Take Back the Night Rally on campus. Under the name Jodaiko, she and several other women from SFTD performed at the rally and began performing at other woman-centered events.

In our interviews, Tamaribuchi never called the dojo's practices sexist or exclusive, but she did point out that when she founded Jodaiko, it became "an opportunity for especially fellow drummers in the Taiko Dojo and other women that were interested in playing the strong parts—but never got the opportunity because all the guys were playing in the Dojo—to get together and play power pieces and not be held back at all." Naomi Guilbert, a core member of Winnipeg's Fubuki Daiko and former SFTD player, remembered performing with Jodaiko during the mid-1990s and told me that a performance at the 1994 West Coast Women's Music Festival was a "brief reprieve from the regular tensions and restrictions" at the SFTD.[26] The dojo seems to have fostered an atmosphere that was open to women but favored men, to the extent that women felt held back in regular rehearsals and excluded from playing the most impressive parts.

Jodaiko was not the only women's taiko group to be formed in response to a need for a women-only space. At about the same time, Canada's first all-women's taiko group, Sawagi Taiko, was formed in 1990 by members of Vancouver-based Katari Taiko (Canada's first taiko group, formed in 1979). In 1989 the female members of Katari Taiko were asked to perform at the Michigan Womyn's Music Festival, a well-known event in lesbian and feminist circles that includes music and camping and is an exclusively female space ("womyn-born-women," in the festival's parlance).[27] Because of this restriction, Katari's male members could not perform at this engagement. According to Eileen Kage, a current Jodaiko member and a member of Katari Taiko at the time, several Katari players (male and female) were uncomfortable with accepting gigs at which only some of the members could perform. Kage remembers the reasoning was that "taiko is for everybody, not just women." Nonetheless, several women from Katari went to Michigan, where their performance was "a big hit."[28] Despite this success and members' excitement about performing at the festival, Katari Taiko decided as a group that if the women wanted to continue performing in spaces restricted to women, they would need to do so under a different name and with their own repertoire. They could use Katari's equipment, but not their songs.

As a result of Katari's policy, several women, including Eileen Kage and Leslie Komori, formed Sawagi Taiko, which, according to its Web site, is a group for "East Asian women living in Canada" that seeks to upend stereotypes of Asians as "mechanical and uncreative" and Asian women as "quiet and demure."[29] Kage remembered that having to create new performance repertoire was like "a blessing in disguise" because it resulted in more creativity, and Komori agreed that they saw it as an "impetus to write a bunch of new songs . . . a lemon into lemonade situation."[30] For reasons unspecified by Kage and Komori, most of Katari's songs were composed by one or two men in the group, but Sawagi was proud of having more of their group members composing than was typical at the time. Although they acknowledged that the situation had been contentious, neither Kage nor Komori spoke of it as a lasting conflict. Both Katari Taiko and Sawagi Taiko still perform in Vancouver, and many of the women who formed Sawagi also continued to perform with Katari.

Jodaiko had begun in 1987, but by the mid-1990s it was performing infrequently. Its 2006 performances constituted a revival of sorts, with a different group of performers and an ersatz home in Vancouver. By that time, both Eileen Kage and Leslie Komori had gained experience performing with various taiko groups in Vancouver: Katari and Sawagi, mentioned above; Uzume Taiko, a trio with fellow taiko player John Greenaway; and LOUD, a trio they formed in 1996 along with guitarist Elaine Stef.[31] After a hiatus from taiko, Kage secured professional development grant funds in 2006 to learn traditional Japanese taiko pieces from Tamaribuchi. Since Tamaribuchi had personal ties in Vancouver, they began to look for places to perform there, along with Komori. When Tamaribuchi formed Jodaiko in 1987, she was essentially a promising beginner with little formal training. In the ten years between the first iteration of the group that played at campus women's events in the 1980s and 1990s and its reemergence in 2006, Tamaribuchi had become a virtuosic, highly trained, and internationally recognized taiko performer. She trained and performed with several professional Japanese groups, including the renowned Ondekoza. In the late 1990s she began entering Japanese taiko competitions, eventually becoming the first American woman to win first place in the All-Japan O-daiko competition in 2001. She had also founded Sacramento Taiko Dan, a group with nonprofit status, a dedicated studio space, and a small paid staff. By this time Tamaribuchi had a reputation of excellence and was a sought-after teacher.

Tamaribuchi's status as a master teacher, her ability to teach traditional reper-toire, and her gender have drawn Jodaiko members to work with her. Kage recalled the time she and Komori spotted Tamaribuchi at a regional taiko gathering in Seattle in 2000: "I remember saying to Leslie, 'Hey that's Tiffany.' Like, [in an awed voice] 'Leslie, that's *Tiffany*.'" Kage stated that, in part, Tamaribuchi's extensive training in Japan had imbued her with an air of authority, as Seiichi Tanaka's and Kenny Endo's experiences in Japan had done for them. She was now a real expert, a sensei, and she was also a woman holding those credentials. Komori said that even though she had been more accustomed to less hierarchical, collectively run taiko groups, she enjoyed learning from and playing with Tamaribuchi, who functions more as a traditional sensei. Komori told me, "I deeply respect her. And I'm grateful for all that she will share." Kristy Oshiro was a teenager performing with Kona Daifukuji Taiko, a youth group associated with a Zen Buddhist temple in Hawai'i, when she met Tamaribuchi. The group's leader, Reverend Tamiya, had invited Tamaribuchi to "teach workshops and provide a strong female taiko player to inspire" the group's many young women. Oshiro and Tamaribuchi kept in touch over the years, and once Oshiro graduated from college, she joined Tamaribuchi's group in Sacramento as well as Jodaiko.[32] Tamaribuchi's visibility as an accomplished taiko player and as a woman have drawn other women players to work with her.

For the 2006 iteration of Jodaiko Tamaribuchi assembled a group of queer Asian women for the performances. As much as Tamaribuchi's status gave her visi-bility, her queerness (or, perhaps, potential queerness) was also legible to those who looked for it or were in the know. Beginning in 2006 Jodaiko began to perform at the queer performance series known at that time as Pride in Art. Although straight-identified women sometimes perform with Jodaiko, the core membership since 2006 has been lesbian and queer-identified women. Tamaribuchi explained that she preferred to feature all queer performers for the Pride in Art event, and since it is easiest to perform a similar lineup there and at Powell Street, the group ended up with an almost exclusively queer membership.[33] There have been times when non-queer and non-Asian performers have participated in Jodaiko's performances. For example, in 2006, when Mu Daiko performed in the Powell Street Festival lineup, four of its members performed with Jodaiko as guest artists (two were queer, two straight; and two were white, two Asian American) at the Pride in Art festival. Most recently, both Nicole Stansbury, who is white and queer-identified, and Sascha Molina, who is black and straight-identified, performed with the group. In addition, one of the members who performed in 2009 identified as gender-nonconforming. Tamaribuchi does not, however, automatically exclude those whose identities fall outside the categories of queer and Asian; rather, she hand-picks players she wants to work with for these particular venues, sometimes including white or straight women and those with non-binary gender identification.

Beyond Jodaiko, queer taiko players have carved out space for themselves at the pre-eminent gathering for taiko players outside Japan, the North American Taiko Conference (NATC), since 2001, but only recently have they done so openly. For several years, taiko players Rachel Ebora and Dane Fujimoto have led a discussion session for queer-identified taiko players called the "Curly Noodle" session. The name is a playful way of describing a queer (that is, not straight) Asian person, and in most years, the session's blurb specifies that the group targets LGBTQ "Asian/Asian American/Asian Canadian participants."[34] The 2005 description indicates that they planned to run concurrent sessions, one for people of color and another for white queer players, with a joint drumming session at the end.[35]

At the 2009 NATC I attended the Curly Noodle session for the first time. The facilitators noted that the fifteen or twenty participants constituted the best turnout so far. (The overall registration for NATC is roughly five hundred to eight hundred people.) They said that previous sessions had attracted only a handful of people. The session was mixed in terms of race, gender, age, and geography and consisted mostly of casual conversation about people's experiences as queer members in taiko groups and ideas for future gatherings. But as Paul Yoon notes, this group had run somewhat under the radar at gatherings as late as 2005, requesting that he as a conference photographer not photograph group members during the session. Members of the group were concerned about their images circulating not only outside taiko circles but in the taiko community as well: "While some stated that they had come out to members of their group," Yoon reports," "others noted that they felt the need to keep quiet about their sexuality because other groups were uncomfortable."[36]

This fear of being seen highlights the extent of the closet and an expectation of homophobia, even among what many taiko players would probably characterize as an accepting and even socially progressive community. At the 2009 meeting the group seemed to be moving in a more "out" direction, with a comfortable and animated atmosphere and with most participants seeming enthusiastic about the suggestion that at the 2011 conference, those interested would perform together as a Curly Noodle group in a conference-wide concert. No NATC was held in 2013, but the Curly Noodle session met again at the 2015 conference, where a small group gathered to discuss a range of issues related to gender and sexual identity. Kristy Oshiro, one of the conveners of the session and a Jodaiko member, told me after the 2015 discussion, "[I]t seems like most groups are very open when it comes to being gay or lesbian or bisexual" but that players who discussed "gender identity, trans issues, and non-monogamy relationships . . . didn't feel ready to come out with that part of their identity yet" for a variety of reasons.[37] Since 2015, trans issues have become much more visible in mainstream media, but it is clear that beyond lesbian, gay, and bisexual taiko players, others who identify under the rubric of queer (whether related to transgender identities or alternative relationship structures) feel more able to discuss their lives in queer-only spaces than within their taiko groups. That the group continues to meet indicates that it provides a useful queer-only space; that their earlier meetings had been held in relative anonymity points again to the presence of—or attendees' vulnerability to the possibility of—homophobia and transphobia within the taiko community, Asian American-Pacific Islander communities, and U.S. and Canadian culture in general.

The venues at which Jodaiko regularly performs (Pride in Art and the Powell Street Festival) highlight their connection to LGBTQ and Japanese Canadian communities. Although Jodaiko has performed at other events in recent years, these two festivals constitute the bulk of their annual performances and to a large extent define the group's existence. At these two festivals, spaces that are centered on Asian Canadian and LGBTQ identity, the group's members are particularly legible as Asian and as queer.

Jodaiko's presence as a visibly queer and Asian taiko group may not constitute a radical form of queer performance, but it is nonetheless significant in the ways it queers North American taiko and performs queer Asian America. Queer Asian American and Pacific Islanders regularly experience racial and sexual harassment and discrimination; and for some, family, religious, or cultural norms prohibit them from living openly as queer.[38] Jodaiko's performances not only constitute a visible, audible presence for queer Asian Americans and Asian Canadians, but the camaraderie they create among themselves is pleasurable for performers as well. In what follows, I demonstrate Jodaiko's queer presence, performances, and pleasures.

HOMO-GENEITY AND ASIAN AMERICAN FEMALE MASCULINITY

On 30 July 2009, I fold up my legs to sit on a tiny plastic child's chair in a small, L-shaped room in the Britannia Ice Arena in East Vancouver. Still dazed from the day of travel between Austin, Texas, and Vancouver, I am glad to simply observe Jodaiko's rehearsal for the weekend's performances and to allow my sweat to dry in the cool air-conditioned room. After greeting me briefly, the Jodaiko members quickly return to the business of rehearsal. Leslie, Eileen, Kristy, and Toyomi, who are all Asian and butch in appearance—that is, they wear their hair short, do not wear makeup, and carry themselves in ways that connote masculinity—stand behind gleaming wooden barrel drums set on polished wooden stands, Tamaribuchi's set of drums on loan from Asano, the renowned Japanese drum makers. They talk through the particulars of the song they are rehearsing. Kristy, an experienced performer, assists the novice Toyomi with her stage presence: "If you look shy, it's going to show. Look cool." Kristy demonstrates shyness with a hunched back and then coolness with a straightened spine and lifted chin. Tiffany bends over a table at the side of the room, writing and revising the lineup for the two upcoming performances. Her dark hair is pulled back into a ponytail that hangs halfway down her back, a change from her usual short-cropped style.

I pluck a piece of grocery-store sushi studded with orange roe from a plastic tray Tiffany pushes toward me and wish I'd brought earplugs to protect my ears from the booming taiko. In the silences between the songs, I am relieved to hear only distant sounds from the hockey rink below: the cool *shhh* of hockey skates against ice, the slap of stick against puck, and the loud drone of a time buzzer marking the periods of a scrimmage. In the cramped space of the rehearsal room, though, it is not only the sound but the percussive vibrations that overwhelm me. For a moment I want to abandon my ethnographic stance and simply perform. I long to swing my left arm into the air as they are doing right now, to clatter out that satisfyingly fast *don ka-ra ka ka, don ka-ra ka ka* on the rim of the drum. As I listen to and watch and feel the rehearsal I begin moving unconsciously with the rhythms, tapping out the phrases on my thighs, letting the chest-rattling drumbeats set my torso in motion. Seeing this, Tiffany hands me a pair of bachi and nods at an open drum, an invitation to play. I struggle to keep up with the rhythms of a song I don't know well, but I am nonetheless happy to play after several years of very little practice and to feel like part of the group. My rusty playing notwithstanding, my racial and gender performance as a white and comparatively feminine woman throws the uniformity of Jodaiko's butch and Asian look into relief.

The members' "homo-geneity," that is, their relatively uniform butchness, makes them legible as queer Asian women. I use the term "homo-geneity" as a playful reference to Lisa Lowe's insistence on the heterogeneity in the category "Asian American." As Lowe asserts, that Asian Americans are "extremely different and diverse among ourselves" disrupts the hegemonic definition of Asian as simply "other" to American[39] Jodaiko's members reflect this very heterogeneity in terms of ethnicity and nationality, but their shared queerness (though each describes her sexuality differently), or homo-geneity (with the emphasis on "homo"), unifies the group. While Asian ethnic diversity is reflected in many ensembles, some groups are organized around more specific identity categories, for example, family connections, temple or church membership, age (for children's groups), or gender. For Jodaiko—organized officially around gender and unofficially around race and sexuality—"homo-geneity" signals coalition, a type of queer belonging, rather than the erasure of difference that the term usually indicates. Moreover, it is the total effect of the group's homo-geneity that allows spectators to see Jodaiko's work as queer performance and as Asian American performance.

Within Jodaiko, butchness and masculinity circulate as both inherent qualities and modes of performance. For the players, "butch" is not a role played purposely against a "femme," as in Sue-Ellen Case's butch-femme aesthetic.[40] Nor do any of these performers strive to pass as men in Jodaiko's shows. Rather, butchness is signaled by short hair, the absence of makeup, and bodily comportment, all of which will be explored in more detail below. When I interviewed Tamaribuchi and asked about Jodaiko and gender performance, she bemusedly noted that she has not intentionally created a butch aesthetic for the group. Nor, in fact, does she cultivate one for herself:

> Everybody identifies *me* as butch. But . . . the thing that makes me butch is the fact that I'm just so not femme. I'm really just so not. I walk into a department store, and I walk through the women's section, and I'm just like nope, nope, nope, nope, nope, nope. Noooo, no, no, no. No. No. And then I walk around and I see, you know, the guy's section and I'm like, okay, I could wear that shirt. I could wear that. And I'd feel comfortable in that.

Throughout our interview, Tamaribuchi repeatedly referred to herself as masculine, both in the way she chooses to look, for example, how she styles her hair and clothing, as well as in her bearing, the way she carries herself. In a discussion of her performances as a competitive o-daiko soloist in Japan, Tamaribuchi described how at one point she constructed a more feminine performance persona for herself after receiving a critique in which the judges felt she performed "too much like a guy . . . an average guy playing." She said

> I had grown my hair out and had gotten this really long, flowy, sequined, you know, outfit, and as I was walking to the concert hall, this guy with a backpack was walking and he looked up and he saw me and he went, "Whoa." [She laughs.] That's the first and only time that's ever happened to me. [She laughs again.] I'm just like, wow. I'm like, "What?" I must've looked like something out of an *anime*, you know. Um, but yeah, . . . and I felt really not so genuine wearing that because it's just not me. Because my bearing is actually not necessarily—like I'm not trying to be masculine. I'm not trying to be butch, but I present that way because it's just kind of the way I move through the world.

The way Tamaribuchi performs with Jodaiko, then, aligns with her gender expression, the way she moves through the world, whereas the sequin-studded brand of femininity she donned for an o-daiko competition she framed as a conscious performance or a construction, one that does not reflect her genuine self (see figure 5.2).

Yet Tamaribuchi also describes an experience that resonates with what David Eng and Alice Hom call the "invisible Asian American lesbian." In the introduction to their edited volume *Q&A: Queer in Asian America*, Eng and Hom argue that race and sexuality are not separate but mutually constitutive phenomena and that the widespread North American cultural perception that Asian men are always already emasculated renders masculine Asian women an impossibility.[41] Commenting on how others perceive her gender performance, Tamaribuchi noted, "All I know is, one of the nicest things about having my hair long is that people don't look at me funny when I go into restrooms. . . . I don't try to have a masculine bearing or presentation, but when my hair is short, all people ever see is 'guy.' " Her comments reveal that without clear markers of femininity (like long hair and sequins), others often assume that she is a man. This perception of Tamaribuchi as male has been borne out when I have made classroom and professional presentations about Jodaiko. Some audience members have trouble assigning Tamaribuchi to the category of female and frequently say they would have assumed that she was male were it not for her very feminine first name. In one instance, this reaction was delivered with disbelief bordering on disgust. While teaching a large lecture class, I screened a video of the whole group performing, and a student sneered, "They're supposed to be *women*?" This young white woman in my classroom saw a group of masculine Asian bodies and could not see them as women. Perhaps her experience and imagination did not include the possibility of lesbians or butch Asian Americans; Eng and Hom might also

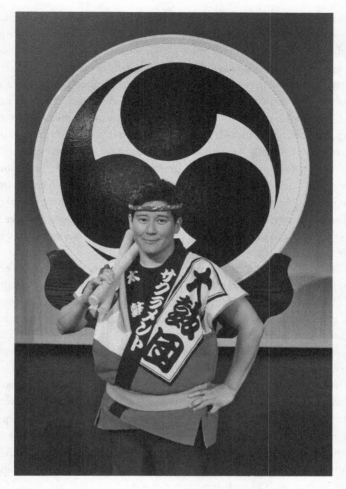

Figure 5.2. Tiffany Tamaribuchi posed in front of the o-daiko. Photo by Katharine Saunders. Used with permission.

argue that when faced with Asian American androgyny, the default position is to see an Asian American male, who is always already feminized or androgynous.

Race, gender, and sexuality are intimately bound up with one another and intersect at the site of Asian masculinity.[42] In order to demonstrate this phenomenon, Eng and Hom open their book with an anecdote: "Consider the following scenario: A short-haired, butch-looking Asian American lesbian is washing her hands in a public women's restroom. A white woman enters. Startled, she checks the sign on the door and then loudly protests, 'This is a women's restroom!' The white woman, assuming that this butch-looking Asian American is a man, claims the restroom as a women's space."[43] The discomfort with which this white woman "saw" a masculine Asian American woman, even in the single-gendered space of a women's restroom, highlights how the "Asian American lesbian goes unseen and unrecognized."[44] Eng and Hom's analysis, and my own, depend to a certain extent on a problematic equation of butchness with lesbianness, but it nonetheless points to the ways assessing sexuality is imbricated with gender normativity.

Onstage, the cumulative effect of Jodaiko members' butch gender performances counters the everyday invisibility of Asian American lesbians that Eng and Hom describe. Stacy Wolf's comments about gender in musical theater also apply to everyday performance: although sexuality and gender expression are two different things, they are "mutually determining." If a woman is alone onstage, not part of a couple, any "unconventional gender performance" can signify her lesbianness. A short haircut, a slightly masculine walk, and un-feminine clothing are just a few examples of the types of codes that one trying to "read queerly" might look for.[45] What constitutes "masculine" and "feminine" is, of course, subjective and dependent on context to a certain extent, yet these gendered choices become ways for audiences to read for sexuality.

Part of Jodaiko's homo-geneity emerges from the very performances of female masculinity that render its members invisible in other spaces. As J. Halberstam writes, "What we call 'masculinity' has always been produced by masculine women, gender deviants, and often lesbians. For this reason, it is inaccurate and indeed regressive to make masculinity into a general term for behavior associated with males."[46] As the anecdote cited above demonstrates, however, it is precisely the intersection between the lesbian's female masculinity *and* her Asianness, always already feminized, that confuses the white woman in Eng and Hom's restroom scenario. That anecdote also raises another issue about visibility and legibility: the very thing that made the Asian American lesbian illegible to this white woman—her butch gender performance—is also the thing that may make her legible *as* a lesbian in queer spaces and contexts. Thus, a range or multiplicity of Asian American female masculinities becomes recognizable as queer bodies in ways a single Asian American woman with a butch appearance might not.

"KOKOROZASHI" AND THE POWELL STREET FESTIVAL

On the first weekend of August each year, white canvas tents dot the perimeter of Vancouver's Oppenheimer Park, where attendees sit on blankets or wander through the Powell Street Festival's varied offerings.[47] Food stalls line one end of the park, offering *yakisoba* (fried noodles), *takoyaki* (octopus fritters), and other Japanese fare. Artisans sell cards, jewelry, t-shirts, and other wares from underneath tents. And in one corner of the park, on the dusty baseball diamond, sits the stage, covered in red-and-white striped canvas, the words POWELL STREET FESTIVAL in bold black-on-white capital letters across the apron of the platform. Throughout the day, musicians, martial artists, and *minyo* (folk) dancers and butoh performers animate this corner of the park as the crowds watch, wander, and move through the festival. The festival has its roots in Japanese Canadian community activism, and its founding marked the hundredth year of Japanese Canadians' presence in Canada, an anniversary that was not lost on its founders.[48] In 1977, socially engaged sansei (third-generation Japanese), some of whom were already involved in providing social services in their community (for example, at the senior center Tonari Gumi), coordinated the first festival, part of a larger effort to reclaim the area surrounding Oppenheimer Park on Powell Street, a neighborhood east of downtown where many Japanese Canadians lived until they were evacuated and interned during World War II. The inaugural festival marked the beginning of what would become a longstanding Vancouver tradition.[49]

I edge my way into the crowd to watch Jodaiko perform "Kokorozashi," one of my favorite pieces. The song is relatively easy to learn, with simple driving patterns interspersed with short improvised solos. Tamaribuchi initially wrote the song as a fun, easy-to-play number for Sacramento Taiko Dan, but it later became an anthem of sorts for several group members who were struggling with breast cancer. Tamaribuchi often dedicates the song to a woman who kept playing taiko throughout chemotherapy and performed at the group's anniversary concert while recovering from a mastectomy, against her doctor's wishes. The piece became emblematic of women's struggles with breast cancer, and as Tamaribuchi told me, it is about "struggle . . . and the choice to not give up and to dare to thrive in the face of adversity."[50]

Although the song's history may be somber, the piece itself bursts with joy. The five drummers begin in a "ready" stance behind a wall of drums lined up across the apron of the stage. Five pairs of legs bend slightly at the knee, feet set wide apart. Ten arms slope toward the ground, mirroring the angle of the legs, bent slightly at the elbow. The drummers seem about to pounce, the bends in their knees and elbows signaling alertness and barely contained energy. Tamaribuchi commands the center drum with quiet authority. She raises one bachi above her head and beats a short introductory riff on the two drums before her, and with a loud "Za!" the other four drummers raise their arms and join her: *DON DON DON DON tsu ten ten ten ten. DON DON DON DON tsu ten ten ten!* They continue pounding out driving unison patterns, their faces alternately showing wide grins and fierce grimaces.

Because each player has been trained in different groups and by different teachers, the group's cohesion does not result from a common technique or years of playing together multiple times each week, as is the case with some groups. Arm angles and stances, even drumbeats, are not necessarily executed with military precision, but the sheer might of their combined energy and the force of seeing five butch Asian American women perform together create a different sort of unity. Short improvised solos pop up among the unison patterns, first a row of short, eight-count solos, then sixteen, and later thirty-two. Kristy keeps her back erect and her chest out as her fast hands fly over the drums. Leslie's arms move fluidly, swinging out in wide arcs as she rocks from foot to foot. Her playing, confident and strong, teeters on the edge of control. As each player takes her solo, her individual playing style emerges, the improvised solos creating room for individual expression within the group dynamic.

As the leader and most virtuosic performer of the group, Tamaribuchi takes her solos last. She begins the solo by playing her own set of drums in the center of the line, as is customary, but quickly moves out of her own space and drums her way down the line, nudging the other players out of their stances. It is a comic bit she has done every time I've seen her perform this number, and it always gets a laugh and cheers from the audience. It could be read as a performance of her status as sensei, a way of playfully using her prerogative to intrude on the other performers' space.[51] But anyone who trains and performs with Tamaribuchi knows that interpretation does not fit her nature. Rather, I read this moment as one in which this powerful and charismatic woman refuses to be contained by the confines of even her own composition. The buoyant and driving energy of the song is uncontainable: by moving into the other women's spaces, she seems to claim this line of drums, the stage, and the festival grounds as a site for abandon, not constraint, for letting go, rather than discipline.

It is not unusual to see such comic bits on a taiko stage. The Japanese touring group Kodo regularly incorporates interpersonal antics into its musical numbers and transitions between songs, as do North American groups San Jose Taiko, San Francisco Taiko Dojo, and numerous others. Here, the moment is flirtatious: as Tamaribuchi drums her way down the line, she exchanges sly smiles with the other women and with us—nothing coy, just enough to draw the audience into her joke. The audience need not know anything about the performers' sexualities to perceive flirtation and charged emotion among women, but the audience must be willing to see women's interactions as potentially queer. Five short-haired women without makeup, wearing uniforms that emphasize the broadness of their shoulders, with body types that range from rail-thin to plump, whose confidence appears unwavering—these qualities open up queer possibilities. Watching the performance, I am unsurprised that, as Tamaribuchi reported, she has quite a few ardent female fans, both those who identify as queer and those who do not. Tamaribuchi queers the taiko stage: the swagger and intensity in her interactions with the other women, her expert command of the drums, and her tomboyish appearance invite a queer gaze.

And she is not alone. After Tamaribuchi's final solo, the group returns to unison drumming, increasing in speed and volume and letting go of precision and control. Faster and louder they drum, and just as the song approaches chaos—*doko doko DON!*—they end the song together, the left bachi pointing skyward and the right pointing to the earth. The five players seem victorious in the electric moments after the song has ended: their arms raised, feet still rooted to the ground, chests heaving with the labor of drumming. Applause and cheers immediately fill the silence: the Powell Street Festival audience is moved in myriad ways by the five queer Asian women onstage, so visibly, audibly, and kinesthetically present.

Homo-geneity, as I have elaborated here, relies primarily on visual cues, but performers' comments also signal that playing with this group of queer Asian women is pleasurable for them as well. Toyomi Yoshida says of the Pride performances:

> I feel like I don't have to hold back as much of who I am. I often feel like I have to do that, living in a straight world. And I think queer audiences appreciate and understand the beauty of strong/butch/non-feminine women. . . . It's a hugely empowering experience to play with other strong, queer women. . . . It's like breathing in fresh air, or having experienced catharsis.[52]

Yoshida's response points to how both audience and performer co-constitute queer performance: the performers by not holding back or by being a version of themselves they may not get to be in everyday life, and the audience by being able to read and enjoy the aesthetics of female masculinity. For Yoshida, at least, this scenario provides not only pleasure but also a profound sense of relaxation. Her references to holding back, to breathing, and to catharsis are doubly valenced. On one hand, they can be understood as aspects of "good" taiko performance in the sense that letting go or playing all out is laudatory. On the other, these words also signal the physical manifestations of being wrapped up, restricted, or closeted—disempowerment, holding one's breath, not feeling the purifying relief of catharsis—that circulate so frequently in narratives of queer life.[53] Jodaiko's performances are more than pleasurable. They queer North American taiko, and they perform queer Asian America. Further, they allow at least one performer to move through the world in ways she otherwise cannot.

The coincidence of the two festivals, LGBT Pride and Powell Street, allows Jodaiko to conveniently play two performances in a short time period, but it also creates a tension for those who want to fully participate in both events. Eileen Kage told me that, historically, Powell Street and Pride happened on different days of the same weekend. In 1996, Pride—a much larger, corporate-sponsored festival— elected to move its day so that it now overlaps with Powell Street. She said, "Many of us who were Asian and queer had to decide what to participate in, negatively [a]ffecting both events (Pride having less Asian visibility and [Powell Street] having less queer visibility)."[54] Tamaribuchi's hope is that Jodaiko's performances continue to bring the queer and Asian Canadian communities together, since both festivals feel like home for the performers. She said, "A lot of people who come to see the [LGBT Pride] show are good friends and part of my network of extended/ chosen family."[55] Given that the Pride performances draw people from queer and Asian Canadian communities, it is unclear whether Tamaribuchi means to single out queer friends as chosen family. Regardless, it is clear that both festivals provide a type of home for Jodaiko performers, whose concerts project homo-geneity for queer, Asian American, and Asian Canadian women. In the following section, I articulate more specifically the erotics of queer spectatorship through a close reading of one of Tamaribuchi's solo numbers.

In contrast to the Powell Street Festival with its outdoor temporary stage in an East Vancouver neighborhood, the Pride in Art queer performance series takes place in a small indoor theater in the heart of downtown Vancouver. In moving from one festival to another, it is not only the geographical and community contexts that shift but also my analytical focus, as I move from considering the collective homogeneity of Jodaiko to the individual performance choices that create the possibility for queer spectatorship in a drum solo by Tamaribuchi. In moving from group playing to a solo number, my focus also shifts to the affective, kinesthetic relation taiko drumming can produce between performer and spectator.

In elaborating my spectatorial relation (even a queerly participatory one) to Tamaribuchi as a performer, I once again risk revealing the Orientalist pleasures wrapped up in taiko performance. Sharon Holland insists, "We can't have our erotic life—a desiring life—without involving ourselves in the messy terrain of racist practice."[56] As a white performer and spectator, I want to mark the tendency, asserted by Richard Dyer, for "white power [to] secure . . . its dominance by seeming not to be anything in particular" and to acknowledge the potentially Orientalist layers of my spectatorship and participation in taiko.[57] As Chapter 2 demonstrates, taiko is often marketed as a centuries-old art form, with ritual and tradition standing in for an Asia that is ancient and unchanging. Eroticized Asian bodies onstage, on the other hand, often call up the taboos associated with Orientalist display and the feminization of Asians as passive sexual objects. My move to mark and complicate the tensions between eroticism and tradition is ultimately a humanizing one. Although there is good reason to be skeptical about language that assumes a transcendental and monolithic human spirit, ethnographer Dorinne Kondo points out that acknowledging the humanity of Asians and Asian Americans—who have often been and continue to be maligned as inhuman in North American contexts—is sometimes "strategically necessary."[58] Moreover, as Celine Parreñas Shimizu asserts, "If we limit understanding of racial sexuality within good or bad, abnormal and normal, or right and wrong we may also limit how we enjoy, appreciate, and more fully understand our own sexuality as Asian/American women."[59] On one level, my attention to the erotic valences of Tamaribuchi's performance gesture to the ways taiko in North America is always already eroticized and racialized, with its focus on bodies that are usually Asian performing for spectators who are often white. Yet, as I hope to demonstrate, taiko performers are seldom passive, and they frequently elicit responses that fall outside typically Orientalist viewing practices. Taiko often situates me and other white performers alongside Asian Americans onstage. My theorizing about queer spectatorship in taiko is, in part, an act of witnessing, my "interactive" response to how race, gender, and sexuality are bound up in the performances that take place both onstage and off.[60]

I sit in the back row, still a good seat in this small venue. It is August 1, 2009, and we are in the overflowing Roundhouse Theater in downtown Vancouver during LGBTQ Pride weekend. Rows of folding chairs have been added in front and at house right to accommodate more people. I estimate that about one-half of the audience is queer: pairs of hand-holding women wearing funky eyeglasses, hefty belts, or short, spiky hair; men wearing Pride T-shirts or standing just close enough together to rule out heterosexuality. Just as performers' stances and gender performances identify them as queer, these audience members' everyday choices of clothing, posture, and physical relationships to others (how they "move together") serve as codes for queer identity. About one-third of the audience appears to be of Asian descent, making this a rare site that brings together queer and Asian Canadian communities. We all sit together in the darkened house waiting for Tamaribuchi's "O-daiko" solo to begin.

To clarify briefly, the term "o-daiko" has several meanings. First, it refers to the drum itself, a large barrel drum, the face of which is usually three to six feet in diameter, that sits sideways atop a tall stand holding the drum four or five feet off the ground. It may also refer to the largest drum onstage. Second, *o-daiko* refers to the way a performer plays this type of drum, usually with his or her back to the audience, facing the drum with arms stretched perpendicular to its face. (An o-daiko workshop, for example, would focus on techniques needed to play drums in this configuration.) And third, "O-daiko" is the title of a the solo piece. This drum is typically associated with male performers and a particular performance of masculine power and aggression.[61] In this concert Tamaribuchi performs the song "O-daiko" in the style of Ondekoza, one of the first professional taiko groups from Japan to tour internationally and with whom Tamaribuchi performed for two years in the mid-1990s.[62] The piece is meant to highlight the virtuosity and stamina of the soloist: depending on the performer, it can last anywhere from about five to twenty minutes. It is also meant to highlight the performer's physique, particularly the musculature of his or her back, and Tamaribuchi's performance follows that tradition (see figure 5.3).

The performance begins long before Tamaribuchi starts to play. The round white face of the drum, perhaps three feet across, glows under the stage lights. Its capacious cylindrical body rests on a tall stand. Tamaribuchi faces the drum, her back to the audience. Her body is compact and fleshy. Her back and arms are mostly bare, except for the thick, criss-crossed straps of her Japanese worker's apron. The ties that hold up her dark blue pants cause the flesh around her hips to bulge gently. Her hair is short, boyish, and dark.[63] In her hands she holds a pair of bachi nearly the length of her arms, their size necessary for producing sound on such a large drum. She settles into a modified martial arts stance, her left leg slightly bent toward the drum and her unbent right leg reaching behind her at a forty-five-degree angle. Her pelvis sinks toward the ground, and for a moment she holds both bachi together in front of her hips, parallel to the floor. She gazes at the drum for a moment, sizing it up like an opponent or a lover, and digs her feet into the ground, rooting herself in the position she will maintain throughout the solo. Then she lifts the bachi above her head and in an instant takes one in each hand. She swings her arms down and

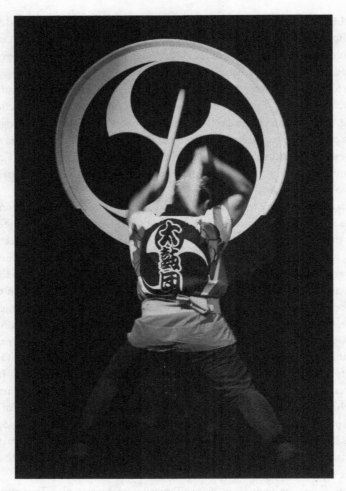

Figure 5.3. Tiffany Tamaribuchi playing the o-daiko. Photo by Katharine Saunders. Used with permission.

apart, matching for a moment the angle of her legs. She tilts her face up toward the drum. Her arms slowly extend out and up, as if tracing an extra-wide snow angel in the air, until they pause above her head—*DO DON*—and break the silence on the skin of the drum.

Even before she begins to play, Tamaribuchi's body is already coded as queer because she defies gender conventions. Tamaribuchi performs masculinity through her bodily stance and the specific way she wears her costume. The *haragake*, or apron, that she wears is a fairly typical taiko costume that both men and women wear, modeled on the kind that a shopkeeper might wear. Taiko players consider it a unisex costume, but it is clearly constructed for men's bodies. Men can wear the haragake over bare chests, but women typically wear sports bras or T-shirts underneath the aprons, which are too stiff and too narrow down the front to fully cover most women's breasts. But Tamaribuchi refuses the security of Spandex and wears nothing under her apron, allowing the slightest curve of her breast to remain visible from the sides. Without anything underneath it, the apron's criss-crossed straps reveal a muscular back and broad shoulders. Rather than highlighting the soft curve of a lower back or delicate neck and shoulders, as might be more typical of women on center stage, Tamaribuchi's costuming highlights the strength in her upper back and the broadness of her shoulders. Still, her body exceeds the costume in a way a man's does not: by allowing her breasts and hips to spill out of the apron, she allows a small suggestion of the feminine to disrupt her otherwise boyish appearance. Tamaribuchi's appearance, more specifically, departs from familiar images of a quiet and demure Asian American femininity evoked by Deborah Wong in her question, "How many of us were taught to keep our knees together and speak softly?"[64] Taiko's movements require Tamaribuchi to take up space in ways that depart from idealized Asian American femininity. Her legs are spread wide apart, and her stance emphasizes the weight of her body. The movement of her arms against the drum highlights the work in her muscles and back, accentuating her strength and endurance. Her costuming, while still allowing her body to be on display, subverts an objectifying gaze by highlighting its strength rather than its shape.

Queer spectatorship of taiko does not begin or end with Jodaiko. In 1975, when Ondekoza introduced "O-daiko" into its concert lineup, it was performed by one of its star drummers, Eitetsu Hayashi. A few days into the performance run at the Espace Pierre Cardin in Paris, fashion designer Cardin suggested a costume change for Hayashi's solo. Rather than wear the several layers of cotton, as did the rest of the group, Hayashi was to wear nothing but *fundoshi*, a simple loincloth worn by sumo wrestlers. The fundoshi covers the man's genitalia but has a G-string effect in the back, leaving his buttocks and the rest of his body exposed. After a few days with Hayashi performing nearly nude, gay men began lining up to see the performances, giving standing ovations each night.[65] Anthropologist Shawn Bender contends that this costuming innovation (now customary for male o-daiko players in some groups) marks the moment when taiko players' bodies, not just the music, became emblematic of virile Japanese masculinity. He writes that the "drummers themselves—or more precisely, their toned, muscular bodies—became a central, if not *the* central, means of expressing their guiding ideology and artistic vision."[66] With this change of costume, the male Japanese body became literally more visible—and legible—not only as a symbol of strength but also as an object of desire, and it was gay male audiences whose presence in the theater declared the costume a success. The gaze, in this instance, was manipulated in a way that was likely meant to capture the attention of straight female audience members, but it appealed to queer spectators, too. This anecdote opens up possibilities for thinking about taiko and queer spectatorship, while it also reminds us of the difficulty of extracting it from a framework of colonialist display in which "othered" bodies are laid bare for the edification of Western audiences.[67] Yet the control and agency with which the drummer performs highlights yet again the tension between performers as objects of consumption and empowered beings in motion. The iconic image of the o-daiko player is a construction of Asian masculinity, as Paul Yoon points out,[68] and Tamaribuchi's reworking of the performance in queer contexts hails queer, lesbian, and feminist possibilities for spectatorship.

In keeping with the tradition set forth by Ondekoza, Tamaribuchi's o-daiko solo is decidedly climactic, even erotic. She plays several slow, even strokes, relishing each arm extension, flexing the muscles in her shoulders and back before quickening her pace and maintaining fast, repeating rhythms. After what seems like several minutes, she shifts to playing short licks on the drum, between which she pauses with her right arm straight above her bowed head. She is teasing her audience with this long series of rhythmic bursts and silent, anticipation-filled poses. She speeds up again, and her stick work becomes impossibly fast as her lower body becomes quieter, more focused on the speed. Tamaribuchi elicits screams and whistles from the audience when she finally transitions back into a powerful frenzy of fast, loud hits to the drum. As the muscles in her arms and back work furiously, the lower half of her body sinks lower, her knees allowing the slightest bounce as she plays. Two women in the front row raise their hands in the air, bouncing in their seats as if in the thrall of an evangelical sermon. Performers yell from offstage, encouraging her as her fast, pounding rhythms reach a climax, then drop in volume and speed for the denouement, a short, slow crescendo. She pulls both arms back—"Soh!"—*DO DON*—and ends the song to the wild applause of the audience.

The potential for queer spectatorship in this performance depends not only on reading Tamaribuchi's costume as queer but also on perceiving the erotics of the drumming, the kinesthetic relation between the audience and the performer. The performance is rich with erotic potential. Given the climactic structure of this largely improvised solo and the way it is meant to excite the audience, it is almost impossible not to invoke sexual imagery—the soft and teasing strokes, the pounding climax—when describing this encounter between two entities, the drummer and the drum, whose bodies and skin make up every taiko performance.

Decoding queer performance depends on reading bodies moving in relation to one another. In this instance Tamaribuchi moves, and her audience moves along with her because it is *moved by* her performance. In a piece in which the performer's back faces the audience, much of the connection between audience and player happens via the drum. The performance is a solo, yet the other overwhelming presence onstage is the drum itself, its round white face looming above Tamaribuchi's head, its loud reverberations filling the chests of everyone inside the theater. Every movement Tamaribuchi makes is toward the drum. Her face and the front of her body, her bachi, and all her energy move upstage toward its expansive surface. Asked about her relationship with the drum, Tamaribuchi said, "It's like having a conversation. It's like arguing or having a fight. It's like making love. It's like dancing. It's surrendering. It's letting go and grooving." When she teaches workshops, she often speaks of the drum in this anthropomorphized fashion as she illustrates the sometimes unpredictable conditions (such as humidity and acoustics) that affect a given drum's feel and sound on a particular day. The drum becomes the site upon which her desire is enacted, played out, and played with. It becomes the vehicle through which desire travels.

The audience's interaction with this performance of desire is where more potential for queer spectatorship emerges. Ramón Rivera-Servera theorizes club dancing as a place where dancers "negotiate their identities and desires" via an "exchange of 'kinesthetic resources.' "[69] Writing specifically about Latina/o gay clubs, Rivera-Servera does not see these spaces as free of structures of power; rather, these are spaces in which identities and relationships are negotiated through dance.[70] As practices involving movement, club dancing and concert taiko performance share a blurring of audience and performer, even if that blurring in taiko is momentary. In the intimate 250-seat Roundhouse Theater, the reverberations of the drumming elicit a kinesthetic response from the audience. In a space that small, every person can feel the drums pounding in their chests and vibrating through the seats. Audiences can experience to some degree what it might feel like to perform, because they, too, can feel the drumming in their bodies; they can't help but participate. The raised hands and bouncing bodies of the women in the front row suggest that they couldn't *not* move along with Tamaribuchi. Moreover, taiko performance can invite spectators to participate by yelling out (in what is called *kiai*) to encourage the drummers during their performances. Usually only audience members who are in the know or who are performers themselves will dare to shout from their seats. But if the performance is exciting enough, as it was in this instance, audience members will respond with screams and catcalls, as well as with applause. Taiko invites instances of embodied, participatory spectatorship that temporarily blur the lines between audience and performer.

What does it mean for an audience to move along with Tamaribuchi, to yell encouragement, and to be moved by her presence onstage? If, to borrow Jonathan Bollen's phrase, "sharing . . . kinesthetic resources"[71] does provide moments when identities and desires can be negotiated and perhaps rearranged, then they also open up space for a queer spectatorship, or an Asian Americanist spectatorship, that does not have to link up with bodily identity. Pointing toward the utopian possibilities of the virtuosic body in performance, Jill Dolan writes, "Audiences often form community around a common present experience of love for a charismatic, virtuosic performer, not necessarily around their desire to be close to him or her, but through the performer, to be pulled into comfortable, more intimate proximity to each other."[72] This is not to say that performance homogenizes its audiences, but it does place them in temporary community together. It may hail Asian American men, queer Asian American women, or straight white women in different ways. But it might ask all spectators, with their multiple and overlapping identities, to respond collectively to queer performance. Whether or not the audience members are queer, they move along with Tamaribuchi in this moment, move along with a woman whose body defies normative femininity, in order to move along with each other in their seats.

As a taiko player, a white spectator, and a queer-identified bisexual woman, when I watch Tamaribuchi's performances, I am moved in several ways. Watching her play makes me want to perform and want to move in the ways she moves. It moves me to yell my encouragement and appreciation for the work the performance requires. I am moved by the history of North American taiko and its anti-racist impulses.[73] I am also moved, even seduced, by Tamaribuchi's charismatic performance, by the fast stick work and the dramatic build of the solo, by her bare back and muscular shoulders. I am moved because I can believe that her performance—her appearance, her costume, her affect—courts *my* gaze. It asks to be seen, heard, and felt as something out of the ordinary. Through her virtuosic performance, her queer gender performance, and the kinesthetic effects of the drumming, Tamaribuchi hails—and momentarily creates—queer spectators.

OTHER POSSIBILITIES

In the years since Jodaiko and Sawagi taiko were formed, other taiko groups and initiatives have formed that actively engage with issues of gender and sexuality. The Toronto-based RAW (Raging Asian Women), formed in 1998, describes itself as "a diverse collective of East and South-East Asian women carrying on the North American taiko drumming tradition and promoting social justice while making music."[74] Its performance and workshops at the 2014 East Coast Taiko Conference at Skidmore College highlighted not only the identitarian focus of the group but also its commitment to an intensive collective-based process and focus on social justice. Their Web site explicitly names queer issues as part of its mission. The Genki Spark, a Boston-based group founded by Karen Young, began in 2010 as a "multi-generational pan-Asian women's arts and advocacy organization that uses Japanese taiko drumming, personal stories, and creativity to build community, develop leadership, and advocate respect for all."[75] The Genki Spark's costumes are lively and eclectic, often featuring bright colors, feminine accessories, and playful makeup, in a departure from North American taiko's tendency toward austere uniformity. Their activities often support social justice issues, including LGBTQ community events. In a talk at the 2015 NATC, Young summed up her thinking about why taiko is effective in building self-esteem for Asian American women and effecting change in the world: "The world needs what we know."

Jodaiko member Kristy Oshiro, in her classes and workshops for queer taiko players, makes explicit what Tamaribuchi has kept an implicit aspect of Jodaiko. In 2014 Oshiro founded a group called Queer Taiko in the Bay Area "for LGBTQQs and allies interested in learning the art of Taiko." One part of an array of performance activities she is involved in, Queer Taiko offers occasional classes and outings in a "safe queer-friendly environment."[76] Each of these groups makes their queerness explicit in mission statements and Web sites listing their values. Jodaiko's queerness, seldom communicated with text, is always present in the flesh and in practice. Each of these groups performs queer Asian America.

My assertion that Jodaiko's performances queer North American taiko is as much about experiencing taiko—and the world—differently as it is about any individual performer's or spectator's self-identification. Jodaiko's performances showcase often marginalized, even "unseen and unrecognized," Asian queer women whose onstage homo-geneity makes them legible to audiences yearning or at least willing to see and hear them. For its early members in particular, Jodaiko let women taiko players experience this art form differently, with expanded possibilities, by allowing them to play power pieces usually reserved for men. And Tamaribuchi's everyday and onstage gender performance undoubtedly invites queer desire and identification via her powerful and often erotic o-daiko solos. In these ways, queering North American taiko is very much tied to identity. And yet not only Asian American women or lesbians enjoy Jodaiko's performances. The performers' virtuosity appeals to a range of spectators, and as they move along together, as we move along with Jodaiko, we may find room to imagine other possibilities.

CHAPTER 6

Conclusion

"This Occasion Needs Context"

From August 8 to August 10, 2017, the first-ever Women and Taiko gathering, a Summer Taiko Institute dedicated to issues related to gender and taiko, was held in the Buddhist Temple of San Diego. The three-day event was led by Karen Young and Tiffany Tamaribuchi, organized by Sascha Molina and Sarah Ayako, and supported by the Taiko Community Alliance. More than forty women, as well as a small number of male and gender-nonconforming participants, spent time at the Buddhist temple thinking, talking, eating, and playing together. The group was multigenerational, multiracial, and multiethnic, and included participants from the United States, Canada, and Europe. It was an intimate gathering that allowed us to talk to one another and hear each other's experiences and perspectives. After about a day and a half of networking, brainstorming, and getting to know one another, we were finally drumming together, doing the thing that connected us in the first place. We had been playing a song called "Joy Bubble," by Tiffany Tamaribuchi, when some of the players formed a circle and started dancing "Tanko Bushi," the popular bon dance, along with the taiko music. The drums were arranged in a large circle, and some of us played a loud, bold *don* pattern on the chu-daiko while others played a faster rhythm on the shime-daiko. We had been playing for some time when the small group set down their bachi and began dancing inside the drummers' circle. It was both collective and spontaneous: people started dancing "Tanko Bushi" because they knew it and because the occasion called for dancing. Soon one or two women joined in with a fue melody, and Tiffany taught us lyrics to sing along with the flute: "I know change is coming / I know change is coming / I know change is coming / Change is coming soon." Drums, flutes, and voices mixed, and bodies moved together. People were smiling, moving from drum to drum, switching parts, stepping in and out of the dance circle, until finally—who knows how much later—we wound down, clapping and sweating.

Later that day, P. J. Hirabayashi gathered us together and said, "This occasion needs context." She told us a story she has told before about a moment in the 1970s when she encountered the joyful spirit of the Asian American movement. As I detail in Chapter 2, Hirabayashi had become politicized as an antiwar college student activist who channeled her anger into protests. Then she saw the Asian American folk duo Chris and Joanne in performance. Chris Iijima, Joanne Miyamoto, and Charlie Chin had released a 1973 album under the name *Grain of Sand* that addressed issues of Asian American identity and social justice. When the duo played the popular obon song "Tanko Bushi" in a rock idiom, their audience of Asian Americans started dancing spontaneously, as we did while playing "Joy Bubble." For P. J., hearing Chris and Joanne's "Tanko Bushi Rock" and seeing the spontaneous dancing it inspired resonated with her as a profound moment in which she recognized that art and joy could mobilize people in ways different from the anger inherent in the rhetoric and protest she experienced in her antiwar activism.

The idea for "Joy Bubble" emerged for Tamaribuchi after the U.S. presidential election of November 2016 when accusations that people were living in their own partisan "bubbles" were circulating in the news and in social media. At a workshop with taiko players in Moab, Utah, she led a practice drill, and a song that could be played at varying skill levels took shape. The name came from Tamaribuchi's sentiment that "if there's going to be a bubble I'm in, I'm going to make it a joy bubble."[1] As the rhythms evolved into a song and as she reflected on the results of the election and the intense racial divides that took center stage in the months that followed, she created lyrics to go with the rhythms. These lyrics, "I know change is coming," were inspired by protest music from the 1960s, in particular, Sam Cooke's "A Change Is Gonna Come." At such a moment, she says, "it was important for people to be grounded in their own truth, given the attacks on 'facts.'"

It is clear that we are in the midst of a new civil rights movement. The shooting death of Michael Brown at the hands of police officer Darren Wilson in Ferguson, Missouri, and the heightened media awareness of subsequent police shootings of black men have resulted in protests and the formation of the activist group Black Lives Matter. All too often, in fact, there is another atrocity to report, for example, the August 2017 conflict that erupted between white supremacist groups and those protesting their hate speech in Charlottesville, Virginia. These highly publicized and carefully staged demonstrations of white supremacist beliefs and the protests denouncing them make clear that deep racial divides persist in the United States. And yet these conflicts also hew closely to a black-white narrative of racism and racial violence, eclipsing the fact that Asian Americans (not to mention Latino/as, Native Americans, and anyone who looks Middle Eastern) are routinely victims of racial violence and live with the effects of everyday, systemic racism.[2] Anger, in other words, is a justified response to these circumstances.

When the participants in the 2017 Women and Taiko gathering played "Joy Bubble" and spontaneously danced "Tanko Bushi" together, the moment resonated with Hirabayashi. As she told the story of Chris and Joanne's "Tanko Bushi Rock," our sweat from "Joy Bubble" was still fresh. Hirabayashi said, "I'm sweating the same sweat." Chris and Joanne's "Tanko Bushi Rock" let its audiences embody an emerging Asian American consciousness and radical politics with joy, connecting (for Japanese Americans, at least) their ethnic heritage with their political imperatives. In a similar way, "Joy Bubble" responded to what many see as a new era of racial consciousness and widespread political unrest, insisting on practicing joy in the midst of justified feelings of anger and despair. Each moment relied on participants' embodied knowledge of a popular obon song; this knowledge is, in part, racial knowledge, one that has a long history in Japanese American communities in particular. Hirabayashi's statement that she was sweating the same sweat points to the ways in which these are not separate historical events but part of an ongoing response to enduring racial and gender inequities in the United States. Playing taiko, dancing "Tanko Bushi," and singing about change together during three days of focusing intensely on issues of gender in and outside of the taiko community allowed us to practice joy amid disheartening, unjust national rhetoric focused on exclusion, misogyny, and white supremacy.

Not all of us who played that day are Asian American, nor American. I cannot speak for any participants' political views, as they surely vary in complex ways, but this was a gathering that encouraged cross-racial intimacy and that generated momentum for social change. The context that P. J. offered underlined the ways in which taiko is deeply enmeshed with Asian American politics, consciousness, and identity. It highlighted, too, how histories of activism (Civil Rights, the Third World movement, feminist movements, the Asian American movement) are not past but rather urgently relevant today. Finally, the spontaneous "Joy Bubble"/"Tanko Bushi" event demonstrated what performance offers in moments of crisis: the opportunity to occupy the same space, breathe the same air, and sweat the same sweat as those around you and the possibility that joy can be harnessed as a political strategy.

This book emerged as a way to explore the many questions that arose from my practice of taiko and from my experience as a white woman in an Asian American performance context. Not all taiko groups frame themselves explicitly as Asian American: some do not need to, since their membership, intentionally or not, is entirely comprised of Asian Americans; other groups have no members who are of Asian descent nor a connection to Asian American communities. What does it mean to perform Asian America in an allegedly post-racial nation whose most urgent racial conflicts are framed as black-white issues? This is one of the queries that frame this book, yet there is a contradiction embedded in the very question. If urgent racial conflicts persist, as they clearly do, then we are not beyond race. Much of this book was written during the Obama presidency. Although it was clear to many that having a black president did not signal the end of racism, in the latter half of 2017 the issues that framed this book seem even more urgent than they did when I began this project. Moreover, the recently emboldened white supremacist movements take positions that are not only anti-black but also anti-immigrant, anti-Semitic, anti-Muslim, anti-woman, and anti-gay. This underscores the need to consider that the question of what it means to perform Asian America must not be narrowly focused on the single category of race.

The preceding chapters have engaged questions of race, gender, and sexuality and their relation to practicing and performing taiko in North America. By now, it should be clear that Asian Americans are not the only ones who perform Asian America, to usher the category into being, and to shape how Asian Americans are viewed, heard, and regarded in the United States. The earliest taiko groups in the nation formed as the very category took shape, and their experiments with group structures, instrument-making and instrumentation, and compositional and choreographic styles were ways of contesting older racial formations and of rehearsing Asian Americanness. Pieces such as P. J. Hirabayashi's "Ei Ja Nai Ka?" that reference and embody Japanese American histories insist that audiences and participants experience these histories—sometimes for the first time—in an embodied way, trying on the gestures and appreciating the labor of immigrant Japanese populations.

But it is not only performers who shape audience reception and perception; marketing and publicity which insist that taiko is part of an ancient and mythic Japan, outreach scenarios that showcase taiko players as exotic talent, and a culture that routinely denies "Americanness" to American citizens of Asian descent all play a role in how Asian America is performed. White and black performers highlight the way Asian Americans are triangulated in just this manner: while they may be considered model minorities in comparison to African Americans (a designation that not only denigrates blacks as the "bad" minority but also glosses over significant differences among Asians in the United States), Asian Americans continue to hover just outside the category "American" (see Chapter 4). Such triangulation is borne out in the experiences of Mu Daiko members, as well as white and black performers in other groups.

Meanwhile, the significance of the Midwest as a site for thinking through Asian American performance cannot be underestimated. The experiences of Mu Daiko members who are Korean adoptees highlight the ways adoptees perform Asian America in complicated ways in Minnesota. The scenarios of recognition that taiko enables among Korean players and audiences demonstrate how performance makes room for changing and critiquing the scenarios of discovery that often accompany Asian American performance. Moreover, the experiences of taiko players in the Midwest suggest, as Josephine Lee writes, that "racial isolation is an experience familiar to many in the Midwest, so much so that it should be thought of as a paradigmatic rather than a peripheral part of Asian American experience."[3] Taiko players may be connected via organizations like the Taiko Community Alliance and at biennial conferences, yet the practice also remains intensely local because so many groups are tied to institutions such as churches, temples, universities, and other arts organizations. Future studies might productively take up focused regional inquiries about taiko in the Southwest, on the East Coast, in Hawai'i, and, of course, in areas beyond the United States and Canada.

As much as my experience in taiko has provided a site for cross-racial intimacy, it has also afforded me and other women expansive models for gender performance and room to follow queer desire. As Chapter 5 demonstrates, the erotic spectatorial experience of taiko offers a foundation for queer readings of Jodaiko's performances, in which players' individual gender performances, costumes, and choreographic choices, particularly at queer festivals, enable such readings. That more groups are forming in order to bring together queer-identified taiko players and perform at key events in LGBTQ communities signals the possibility for coalition across queer and Asian American communities.

Beyond the groups and individuals who form the basis of this book, the taiko scene is changing faster than I can write. Rather than expand on what would be an exhaustive list of new directions in the form, I close by returning to the Women and Taiko gathering. During the three days we spent together, I heard several Asian American women describe taiko as something that radically transformed the way they understood themselves. For some, this happened in the 1970s, and for others, it happened much later. I observed male-identified participants listening and learning from women's experiences, a model I hope others will follow. I heard cross-generational discussions about gender fluidity and about what feminism means to them. And I heard multiple perspectives, questions, and disagreements about what the future should bring for taiko. In other words, it was not a homogenous, single-minded group. But it was a group that, thanks in large part to Karen Young's facilitation skills, learned a great deal from one another's experiences.

As we drummed the rhythms of "Joy Bubble" and danced "Tanko Bushi," we sang about change. Embodied repertoires, in Diana Taylor's formulation, harbor the hope of changing familiar (and often oppressive) scenarios.[4] What changes can future taiko practices body forth? What cultural memory will our performances transmit to future practitioners? What sweat will we be sweating together? Despite the diversity among us, it would have been difficult for participants to leave the Women and Taiko gathering without a sense of how inextricably enmeshed taiko is with Asian American histories. Every player should seek out and listen to the histories and cultural politics of taiko, not just as a product of Japan but as something very much informed by Asian American cultural politics, by gendered dynamics, and even by sexuality. I will be pleased if this book offers an avenue into that understanding. Moreover, I hope it offers others the opportunity to reflect on, question, expand upon, and challenge the ideas set forth here and to take pleasure in taiko not only as a practice, but as a site for critical inquiry. Finally, I hope this book offers taiko players and other performance-makers strategies for engaging the cultural politics of their practice, whether in festivals, gymnasiums, rehearsal rooms, theaters, or the myriad other places in which they get to move and make noise.

APPENDIX A
List of Interviews by the Author

Amanda [surname withheld]. Email interview. July 1, 2017.

Amundson, Gregg. Personal interview. June 27, 2009.

Ellsworth, Jeff. Personal interview. June 25, 2009.

Endo, Kenny. Personal interview. March 7, 2014.

Gorton, Rachel. Personal interview. June 27, 2009.

Guilbert, Naomi. Email interview. September 22, 2009.

Kage, Eileen. Personal interview. July 31, 2009.

Ko, Su-Yoon. Email interview. June 15, 2016.

Komagata, Faye and Shuji Komagata. Personal interview. March 7, 2014.

Komori, Leslie. Personal interview. August 2, 2009.

Kuniyoshi, Susie. Personal interview. June 19, 2009.

Lee, Heewon. Personal interview. June 18, 2009.

Molina, Sascha. Personal interview. June 13, 2015.

Okada, Alan. Personal interview. October 10, 2015.

Oshiro, Kristy. Email interview. February 2, 2010.

San Jose Taiko members (Yurika Chiba, P. J. Hirabayashi, Roy Hirabayashi, Franco Imperial, Meg Suzuki, and Wisa Uemura), personal interview, September 29, 2009.

Shiomi, Rick. Personal interview. June 18, 2009.

Shiomi, Rick. Personal interview. August 8, 2009.

Shiraishi, Iris. Personal interview. June 19, 2009.

Sotelo, Tanis. Email interview. June 6, 2017.

Stansbury, Nicole. Personal interview. June 12, 2015.

Tamaribuchi, Tiffany. Personal interview. October 12, 2009.

Wells, David. Email interview. November 16, 2015.

Weiner, Adam. Personal interview. June 11, 2015.

Weir, Jennifer. Personal interview. June 28, 2009.Yoshida, Toyomi. Email interview. January 21, 2010.

Youngblood, Shereen. Personal interview. June 29, 2017.

Zdrazil, Al. June 25, 2009.

APPENDIX B

List of Life History Interview Transcripts Consulted

Life History Interview Transcripts, courtesy of the exhibition *Big Drum: Taiko in the United States*, Hirasaki National Resource Center, Japanese American National Museum, 369 East First Street, Los Angeles, CA 90012.

Abe, George. Life History Interview. December 10, 2004.
Baba, Russell. Life History Interview. January 24, 2005.
Banks, Dennis. Life History Interview. February 1, 2005.
Hirabayashi, P. J. Life History Interview. January 26, 2005.
Hirabayashi, Roy. Life History Interview. January 26, 2005.
Kodani, Reverend Masao. Life History Interview. December 3, 2004.
Mercer, Jeanne. Life History Interview, January 24, 2005.

NOTES

PREFACE

1. Judith Hamera, *Dancing Communities: Performance, Difference, and Connection in the Global City* (New York: Palgrave Macmillan, 2007), 40–41.
2. Ibid., 54.
3. Jeanne Mercer, Life History Interview, January 24, 2005, Life History Interviews (transcripts), *Big Drum: Taiko in the United States* exhibition, Hirasaki National Resource Center, Japanese American National Museum, 369 East First Street, Los Angeles, CA 90012 (hereinafter HNRC/JANM archive).
4. Matthew Rahaim, *Musicking Bodies: Gesture and Voice in Hindustani Music* (Middletown, CT: Wesleyan University Press, 2012), 1.
5. Ibid.
6. See Angela K. Ahlgren, "A New Taiko Folk Dance: San Jose Taiko and Asian American Movements," in *Contemporary Directions in Asian American Dance*, ed. Yutian Wong (Madison: University of Wisconsin Press, 2016), 29–61; Masumi Izumi, "Reconsidering Ethnic Culture and Community: A Case Study on Japanese Canadian Taiko Drumming," *Journal of Asian American Studies* 4 (2001): 35–56; Paul Jong-Chul Yoon, "'She's Really Become Japanese Now!': Taiko Drumming and Asian American Identifications," *American Music* (Winter 2001): 422–424.
7. For demographic information, see "Taiko in the USA and Canada: Key Findings from the Taiko Census 2016." Prepared by Kate Walker on behalf of the Taiko Community Alliance. https://taikocommunityalliance.org/events/census/, accessed December 2, 2017. The work is released under a Creative Commons–Attribution Share-Alike 4.0 International license. For discussions of the feminist potential of taiko, see Deborah Wong, "Taiko and the Asian/American Body: Drums, *Rising Sun*, and the Question of Gender," *World of Music* 42, no. 3 (2000): 67–78; Izumi, "Reconsidering Ethnic Culture," 44–46.
8. Paul Jong-Chul Yoon, "Asian Masculinities and Parodic Possibilities in Odaiko Solos and Filmic Representations," *Asian Music* (Winter–Spring 2009): 100–130. Yoon establishes the ways taiko, especially the style of playing the large *o-daiko*, is coded as masculine in both Japanese and American contexts. He contextualizes his discussion of Japanese o-daiko playing within the post–World War II era in Japan.
9. Deborah Wong, "Moving: From Performance to Performative Ethnography and Back Again," in *Shadows in the Field: New Perspectives for Fieldwork in Ethnomusicology*, 2nd ed., ed. Gregory Barz and Timothy J. Cooley (New York: Oxford University Press, 2008), 79, italics in original.
10. I borrow the term "witness" from dance scholar Ann Cooper Albright to invoke a "responsiveness, a response/ability of the viewer toward the performer" rather than a consuming, one-way gaze. Ann Cooper Albright, *Choreographing Difference: The Body and Identity in Contemporary Dance* (Middletown, CT: Wesleyan University Press, 1997), xxii.
11. Hamera, *Dancing Communities*, 1.

CHAPTER 1

1. The Taiko Census is a project of TCA. The first census was conducted in 2013, and another was conducted during May 2016. See "Taiko Census," https://taikocommunityalliance.org/events/census/, accessed December 4, 2017.

2. Hamera, *Dancing Communities*, 1 (see preface, n1).

3. Ramón Rivera-Servera, *Performing Queer Latinidad: Dance, Sexuality, Politics* (Ann Arbor: University of Michigan Press, 2012), 34.

4. Deborah Wong, *Speak It Louder: Asian Americans Making Music* (New York: Routledge, 2004), 203.

5. Heidi Varian, *The Way of Taiko* (Berkeley, CA: Stone Bridge Press, 2005), 16.

6. Paul Jong-Chul Yoon critiques a similar history of Japanese taiko in a documentary about the Japanese performing group Kodo. See Yoon, "'She's Really Become Japanese Now!'" (see preface, n6). The documentary *The Spirit of Taiko* (dir. Steven Dung, Diane Fukami, and Gayle K. Yamada, DVD, Bridge Media, 2005), also draws on these mythologies.

7. Yoon, "'She's Really Become Japanese Now!'" 417–438.

8. While I and other taiko scholars have emphasized the ways in which taiko is largely a contemporary form (a move that attempts to divorce taiko from Orientalist views of its association with an "ancient" Japan as described above), some players do study and perform traditional drum musics of Japan as part of, or as a supplement to, their taiko practice. See ibid.; Anna Viviano, "Made in Japan: Kumi-daiko as a New Art Form" (PhD diss., University of South Carolina, 2013). Although taiko instruments from the festival traditions initially came to the United States with the first wave of Japanese immigrants in the 1900s, the contemporary tradition did not take the same diasporic route but, rather, was taken up by sansei, or third-generation Japanese Americans, as a way to connect to their ethnic roots. See D. Wong, *Speak It Louder*, 203; for a thorough explanation of the instrumentation, costuming, and other material and practical aspects of taiko in the United States, see Mark Tusler, "Sounds and Sights of Power: Ensemble Taiko Drumming (Kumi Daiko) Pedagogy in California and the Conceptualization of Power" (PhD diss., University of California at Santa Barbara, 2003).

9. According to Shawn Bender, this group changed leaders and names several times early in its history. See Shawn Bender, *Taiko Boom: Japanese Drumming in Place and Motion* (Berkeley: University of California Press, 2012) 18–19.

10. For a detailed account of the first Japanese taiko ensembles, see ibid., 48–104.

11. Jennifer Milioto Matsue, "Drumming to One's Own Beat: Japanese Taiko and the Challenge to Genre," *Ethnomusicology* 60, no. 1 (Winter 2016): 23.

12. The 2013 conference was postponed as conference organizers strategized about how to support future gatherings, and a conference was held in Las Vegas, Nevada, in June 2015. Further attention to the organizational shift from the JACCC to the TCA is beyond the scope of this book, but more information about the TCA and the North American Taiko Conference can be found at www.taikocommunityalliance.org.

13. Matsue, "Drumming," 23.

14. William Wei, *The Asian American Movement* (Philadelphia: Temple University Press, 1993), 2.

15. Glenn Omatsu, "'Four Prisons' and the Movements of Liberation: Asian American Activism from the 1960s to the 1990s," in *Asian American Studies: A Reader*, ed. Jean Yu-Wen Shen Wu and Min Song (New Brunswick: Rutgers University Press, 2000), 168.

16. Wei, *Asian American Movement*, 13–15. See also Omatsu, "'Four Prisons,'" 165, and Diane Fujino, "Race, Space, Place and Political Development: Japanese-American Radicalism in the 'Pre-Movement' 1960s." *Social Justice* 35, no. 2 (2008): 70.

17. Wei, *Asian American Movement*, 45.

18. See Laura Pulido, *Black, Brown, Yellow, and Left: Radical Activism in Los Angeles* (Berkeley: University of California Press, 2006), 54. In an interview for the 2005 exhibit titled "Big Drum" at the Japanese American National Museum, Kodani said he lived in black neighborhoods in Los Angeles. He recalls speaking "black" English with his peers and feeling in many ways more akin to his black peers than to other Japanese Americans. Similarly, Roy Hirabayashi, a founder of San Jose Taiko, described growing up in a primarily black neighborhood of Oakland and observing Black Panther members patrolling the area. Many sansei not only were informed politically by growing up in black neighborhoods but also attributed their musical tastes to listening to Afro-Cuban styles. Reverend Masao Kodani, Life History Interview, HNRC/JANM archive, December 3, 2004; Roy Hirabayashi, Life History Interview, HNRC/JANM archive, January 26, 2005.

19. Steve Louie, "When We Wanted It Done, We Did It Ourselves," in *Asian Americans: The Movement and the Moment* (Los Angeles: UCLA Asian American Studies Center Press, 2001), xix.

20. Wei, *Asian American Movement*, 64.

21. Ibid., 66.

22. Ibid., 65.

23. Yoshimi Kawashima, "GIDRA: The Voice of the Asian American Movement," Discover Nikkei Web site, http://www.discovernikkei.org/en/journal/2012/1/12/gidra/, accessed January 12, 2012.

24. Esther Kim Lee, *A History of Asian American Theatre* (Cambridge: Cambridge University Press, 2006), 26–27.

25. Ibid., 29. They protested yellowface casting in *Here's Where I Belong* and *The King and I* on Broadway in 1968, and in 1970 they protested the casting of *Lovely Ladies, Kind Gentlemen* at Lincoln Center.

26. Wong, *Speak It Louder*, 195–196.

27. "Taiko in the USA and Canada."

28. See Claire Jean Kim, "The Racial Triangulation of Asian Americans," *Politics & Society* 27, no. 1 (March 1999): 105–138.

29. Priya Srinivasan, *Sweating Saris: Indian Dance as Transnational Labor* (Philadelphia: Temple University Press, 2011), particularly chap. 3, "Archival Her-stories: St. Denis and the *Nachwalis* of Coney Island," 67–92; Yutian Wong, *Choreographing Asian America* (Middletown, CT: Wesleyan University Press, 2010), 43–51.

30. "About," San Francisco Taiko Dojo Web site, http://www.sftaiko.com/tanaka-1/, accessed March 19, 2015.

31. Dennis Banks, Life History Interview, HNRC/JANM archive, February 1, 2005.

32. According to performance studies scholar Hideyo Konagaya, Tanaka's status "has been kept intact through his professional manipulations, including the dramatization of his legendary image as the founder of North American Taiko." See Hideyo Konagaya, "Taiko as Performance: Creating Japanese American Traditions," *Japanese Journal of American Studies* 12 (2001): 119.

33. Mark Tusler ("Sounds and Sights of Power") has written the most detailed account of Tanaka's history as a taiko player. For more information on Osuwa Daiko and Oguchi Daihachi, see Bender, *Taiko Boom*.

34. Although Rebecca King cites 1968 as the first year the festival was held, other sources indicate that 1967 was its inaugural year. Still, sites such as http://www.nccbfqueenprogram.org/past-cherry-blossom-courts.html list 1968 as the first annual festival while also listing 1967 as the beginning of the festival. In any case, it seems that Tanaka attended a festival in 1967 as a spectator and returned the following year as a performer. Rebecca Chiyoko

King, "Multiraciality Reigns Supreme? Mixed-Race Japanese Americans and the Cherry Blossom Queen Pageant," *Amerasia Journal* 23, no. 1 (1997): 116.

35. See King, "Multiraciality"; see also Benjamin Pachter, "*Wadaiko* in Japan and the United States: The Intercultural History of a Musical Genre," PhD diss., University of Pittsburgh, 2013, 198.

36. Tusler, *Sounds and Sights*, 133–134.

37. Tusler pinpoints this shift in 1980, whereas Pachter points out that "Dojo" appeared as part of the group's name earlier 1977. See Tusler, *Sounds and Sights*, 139; Pachter, "Wadaiko," 209.

38. Pachter, "Wadaiko," 200–201.

39. According to Pachter, Tanaka and the other drummers received lessons and equipment from a group of Japanese musicians on tour in the United States. Included among the performers were members of Sukeroku Taiko (a group of star drummers from Tokyo) and Ishizuka Yutaka, who would later become known by his *natori* (stage name) Mochizuki Saburo. It was shortly after this visit that Tanaka returned to Japan to study with Oguchi Daihachi, who by this time had agreed to teach him, albeit secretly. The connections Tanaka made with Sukeroku Taiko members and with Ishizuka/Mochizuki while they were in California not only allowed him training he had been unable to access in Japan but also gave Tanaka access to their professional-grade instruments, which they were unable to ship home to Japan. See ibid., 198–199.

40. Samuel Fromartz, "Anything but Quiet," *Natural History* (March 1998), n.p.

41. See Fujino, "Race, Space, Place."

42. Kodani, Life History Interview.

43. Abe describes being involved with the Amerasia Bookstore in Los Angeles and socializing with people who published *Gidra*; both were associated with the Yellow Power movement. He also had been involved with Oriental Concern, a consciousness-raising group that focused on identity and "model minority" stereotypes. See George Abe, Life History Interview, HNRC/JANM archive, December 10, 2004.

44. Susan Asai, "Horaku: A Buddhist Tradition of Performing Arts and the Development of Taiko Drumming in the United States," *Selected Reports in Ethnomusicology* 6 (1985): 163–164.

45. Kodani, Life History Interview.

46. It is also possible that some of them saw the taiko performance that was part of the opening ceremony of the 1964 Tokyo Olympics. See Hideyo Konagaya, "Performing the Okinawan Woman in Taiko: Gender, Folklore, and Identity Politics in Modern Japan" (PhD diss., University of Pennsylvania, 2007).

47. The Japanese American National Museum site hosts a helpful timeline and photo gallery of early taiko groups in the United States: http://www.janm.org/exhibits/bigdrum/gallery/. The Web site Discover Nikkei also hosts a page on taiko: http://www.discovernikkei.org/en/taiko/.

48. Omatsu, "'Four Prisons,'" 184. For a concise narration of post-1965 Asian America, see also Erika Lee, *The Making of Asian America: A History* (New York: Simon & Schuster, 2015), 283–313.

49. "About Stanford Taiko," http://web.stanford.edu/group/stanfordtaiko/cgi-bin/about.php, accessed August 14, 2016; Linda Uyechi, pers comm, Jan 18, 2018.

50. See, for example, Eiichiro Azuma, *Between Two Empires: Race, History, and Transnationalism in Japanese America* (Oxford: Oxford University Press, 2005); Mae M. Ngai, *Impossible Subjects: Illegal Aliens and the Making of Modern America* (Princeton, NJ: Princeton University Press, 2004), among many others.

51. Karen Shimakawa, *National Abjection: The Asian American Body Onstage* (Durham: University of North Carolina Press, 2002), 57.

52. Josh Kun, *Audiotopia: Music, Race, and America* (Berkeley: University of California Press, 2005), 13.

53. My thinking about "Asian America" as a racial formation is informed by Omi and Winant's understanding of racial formation as a set of historically situated processes, policies, and attitudes through which categories of race are made and remade. Omi and Winant, *Racial Formation in the United States* (New York: Routledge, 1986), 55.

54. D. Wong, *Speak It Louder*, 11; Grace Wang, *Soundtracks of Asian America: Navigating Race through Musical Performance* (Durham, NC: Duke University Press, 2015), 4.

55. Richard Schechner, *Performance Studies: An Introduction* (London: Routledge, 2002), 191; Christopher Small, *Musicking: The Meanings of Performing and Listening* (Middletown, CT: Wesleyan University Press, 1998), 9.

56. My thinking about Asian America as something that comes into being through repeated performance is informed by Judith Butler's theory about gender as performativity. See Butler, "Performative Acts and Gender Constitution: An Essay in Phenomenology and Feminist Theory," *Theatre Journal* 40, no. 4 (December 1988): 519–531, and by Gary Okihiro's notion that "Japanese American" takes shape through doing. Gary Okihiro, "Acting Japanese," in *Japanese Diasporas: Unsung Pasts, Conflicting Presents, and Uncertain Futures*, ed. Nobuko Adachi (New York: Routledge, 2006), 195.

57. D. Wong, *Speak It Louder*, 13.

58. See Lisa Lowe, *Immigrant Acts: On Asian American Cultural Politics* (Durham, NC: Duke University Press, 1996), 72; and Shimakawa, *National Abjection*, 3.

59. Grace Wang, *Soundtracks of Asian America* (Durham, NC: Duke University Press, 2015), 19.

60. Yutian Wong, "Introduction," in *Contemporary Directions in Asian American Dance*, ed. Yutian Wong (Madison: University of Wisconsin Press, 2016), 10.

61. Y. Wong, *Choreographing Asian America*, 39.

62. Wong also makes this observation in her edited volume, *Contemporary Directions in Asian American Dance*, 5–6.

63. Rahaim, *Musicking Bodies*, 1 (see preface, n4).

64. Alan Okada, personal interview, October 10, 2015.

65. Other works concerning taiko omit women, as well. The documentary *Spirit of Taiko* features Seiichi Tanaka, Kenny Endo, and Masato Baba as three generations of taiko players in the United States. Although both of Baba's parents are well-known taiko players who trained with Tanaka and run their own group in Mount Shasta, this film constructs a genealogy of taiko greats in which the form is passed down from one man to another.

66. See Yoon, "Asian Masculinities," 100–130 (see preface, n8); and Bender, *Taiko Boom*, 6.

67. D. Wong, "Taiko and the Asian/American Body," 74–75 (see preface, n7).

68. See Yoon, "Asian Masculinities."

69. Erika Lee (*Making of Asian America*, 309–311) locates the beginning of an Asian American LGBT movement in 1979.

70. Rivera-Servera, *Performing Queer Latinidad*, 27.

CHAPTER 2

1. A YouTube clip titled "Ei Ja Na Kai—Post Taiko Jam Jam 2009" from the North American Taiko Conference in 2009, posted by kaukadj on August 20, 2009, can be seen here: https://www.youtube.com/watch?v=c8Z7a4e5sBg, accessed August 15, 2016.

2. P. J. Hirabayashi, who created the piece, teaches "Ei Ja Nai Ka?" in workshops. With her permission, groups are allowed to perform the piece and teach it to their own members.

3. "Obon" refers to a late-summer festival that honors the dead. These events are common throughout Japan and the Japanese diaspora. Cherry blossom festivals are celebrated in the spring.

4. In such a workshop we learn the basic drum rhythms, the call-and-response chants, and the dance moves. There are other elements to the song—such as a melody with lyrics and other auxiliary percussion parts—that could be learned in further workshops.

5. "Taiko in the USA and Canada" (see preface, n7).

6. See, for example, Roy Hirabayashi, Life History Interview (see Chapter 1, n18).

7. For more on the Asian American movement, see Yen Le Espiritu, *Asian American Panethnicity: Bridging Institutions and Identities* (Philadelphia: Temple University Press, 1992), 25, 31–32; Michael Liu et al., *The Snake Dance of Asian American Activism: Community, Vision, and Power* (Lanham, MD: Lexington, 2008); Wei, *Asian American Movement* (see Chapter 1, n14).

8. See, for example, George Abe, Life History Interview (see Chapter 1, n43).

9. Liu et al., *The Snake Dance*, xv.

10. Ibid.

11. P. J. Hirabayashi and San Jose Taiko, handout, unpublished score (1994), distributed in the "Ei Ja Nai Ka?" workshop at the 2009 North American Taiko Conference.

12. Re-membering, for Thiong'o, is a set of practices deployed by African writers in a "quest for wholeness" after the dis-memberment of Africa under colonialism. He writes, "Creative imagination is one of the greatest of re-membering practices. The relationship of writers to their social memory is central to their quest and mission. Memory is the link between the past and the present, between space and time, and it is the base of our dreams." Ngugi wa Thiong'o, *Something Torn and New: An African Renaissance* (New York: Basic Civitas Books, 2009), 39. My thanks to Rachel Wishkoski, who pointed out that my use of "re-membering" resonated with that of Thiong'o.

13. Charlotte Canning, "Feminist Performance as Feminist Historiography," *Theatre Survey* 45, no. 2 (November 2004): 230.

14. Ibid.

15. Roy Hirabayashi, Life History Interview.

16. See the National Endowment for Arts' National Heritage Fellowship page, http://arts.gov/honors/heritage.

17. Jennie Knapp, "Ensemble's Mix of Drumming, Dance Thrilling," *Richmond Times-Dispatch*, March 2, 1999, D6.

18. D. Wong, "Moving," 76 (see preface, n9).

19. Roy Hirabayashi and P. J. Hirabayashi are the only two current members of San Jose Taiko who were also part of the group's formative years. Other founding members were not interviewed either by me or the JANM staff during the *Big Drum* exhibit. My analysis, therefore, is based largely on the memories of these two individuals.

20. Schechner, *Performance Studies*, 191 (see Chapter 1, n55); Small, *Musicking*, 9 (see Chapter 1, n55).

21. Rahaim, *Musicking Bodies*, 1 (see preface, n4).

22. Small, *Musicking*, 8.

23. Wisa Uemura, email to the author, March 29, 2012.

24. Elin Diamond, "Introduction," in *Performance and Cultural Politics*, ed. Elin Diamond (New York: Routledge, 1996), 1.

25. Gary Okihiro, "Acting Japanese," 195.

26. Roy Hirabayashi, Life History Interview.

27. For a further discussion of Japanese taiko's multiple influences, see Bender, *Taiko Boom* (see Chapter 1, n9).

28. P. J. Hirabayashi, Life History Interview, January 26, 2005.

29. Joni L. Jones, "Performance Ethnography: The Role of Embodiment in Cultural Authenticity," *Theatre Topics* 12, no. 1 (2002): 14.

30. Wei, *Asian American Movement*, 11.

31. P. J. Hirabayashi, Life History Interview.

32. San Jose Taiko members (Yurika Chiba, P. J. Hirabayashi, Roy Hirabayashi, Franco Imperial, Meg Suzuki, and Wisa Uemura), personal interview, September 29, 2009 [hereafter "San Jose Taiko members, personal interview"].

33. See E. Lee, *Making of Asian America*, 309 (see Chapter 1, n48); William Wei, *Asian American Movement*, 76–77. Thanks to Jonathan Chambers for pointing out that San Jose Taiko managed to succeed with regard to issues of gender where many New Left groups had failed.

34. San Jose Taiko members, personal interview.

35. Yuji Ichioka, quoted in Eiichiro Azuma, "Editor's Introduction: Yuji Ichioka and New Paradigms in Japanese American History," in Yuji Ichioka, *Before Internment: Essays in Prewar Japanese American History*, ed. Gordon H. Chang and Eiichiro Azuma (Stanford: Stanford University Press, 2006), xvii.

36. Taikoprojects's theater-taiko piece *Pioneers*, for example, interweaves monologues with performances of these three groups' most popular songs.

37. Eiichiro Azuma, *Between Two Empires: Race, History, and Transnationalism in Japanese America* (Oxford: Oxford University Press, 2005), 91.

38. See Izumi, "Reconsidering Ethnic Culture," 35–56 (see the preface, n6).

39. Jere Takahashi, *Nisei/Sansei: Shifting Japanese Identities and Politics* (Philadelphia: Temple University Press, 1997), 2. This sentiment was echoed in the interviews I conducted and the oral history transcripts I read.

40. Ibid., 85.

41. Ibid., 197–200.

42. The search for Japanese cultural activities by sansei is a prevalent theme in the interviews I conducted as well as the oral history transcripts I read. For a thorough exploration of generational dynamics between nisei and sansei, see ibid.

43. P. J. Hirabayashi, Life History Interview.

44. San Jose Taiko members, personal interview.

45. P. J. Hirabayashi, email to the author, June 17, 2010.

46. *Big Drum: Taiko in the United States*, dir. Akira Boch, Sojin Kim, and Masaki Miyagawa, DVD, Frank H. Watase Media Arts Center, Japanese American National Museum, 2005.

47. Rachel Wishkoski, "To Become Something New Yet Familiar": Remembering, Moving, and Re-membering in Seattle Buddhist Church's Bon Odori Festival." MA thesis, Ohio State University, 2014, 1.

48. Warabi-za's Web site indicates that the group "prides itself in depicting contemporary society through the arts." In addition to seven performing troupes, Warabi-za runs the Folk Arts Research Center, which houses thousands of folk songs and dances; See "Warabi-za," http://www.warabi.jp/english/aboutus.html, accessed August 15, 2016.

49. The general meaning of the chant is "Isn't it good?" "Ready, ready!" "Isn't it good?" "Ready, ready, here we go!" In taiko, "So-re!" is often shouted just before beginning a number, something like "Five, six, seven, eight!" or "Ready, and!" in dance. Similarly, "Yoi-sho!" has no particular meaning but keeps time.

50. Ronald Takaki, *Strangers from a Different Shore: A History of Asian Americans*, rev. ed. (Boston: Little, Brown, 1998), 221–223.

51. Yoko Fujimoto, "'Ei Ja Nai Ka?' Lyrics to Accompany Dance," unpublished manuscript, 2001. Just as the dance is gestural, using simple stylized movements to convey its meanings, the song lyrics use a spare poetic style to create a progress narrative moving from migration to labor to progress to celebration. The lyrics (different from the call-and-response chanting) were added later in the song's development. The lyrics are written and sung in Japanese, with only a few English phrases throughout, so only audiences with an understanding of the Japanese language would have total access to the layers of meaning

as they watch a performance. San Jose Taiko has provided me with two translations, one that is (in P. J. Hirabayashi's words) more "literal" and another that is "poetic." Since my analysis depends on the general meaning of the song rather than a close textual reading, I refer to the poetic translation here. The song is composed of four verses, with the refrain "Ei Ja Nai Ka?" [Isn't it good?] repeated in the second and third lines of each verse.

52. Takaki, *Strangers from a Different Shore*, 44. As Takaki writes, many issei "saw themselves as *dekaseginin*—laborers working temporarily in a foreign country."

53. San Jose Taiko members, personal interview.

54. Fujimoto, "Lyrics to Accompany Dance." For the sake of simplicity, I have omitted the Japanese translation of lines 1, 4, and 5. It is the Japanese that is actually sung in performance; my purpose is to illuminate meanings for an English-speaking audience. Like "Grandma" and "Grandpa" in the first verse, "Railroad" and "Steam Engine" are pronounced with extra syllables: "Suti-ime En-gine" and "Ra-il ro do."

55. Takaki, *Strangers from a Different Shore*, 182–185.

56. Ichioka quoted in Azuma, "Editor's Introduction," xvii.

57. Takaki, *Strangers from a Different Shore*, 180–197.

58. Ibid., 186.

59. Ibid., 191.

60. San Jose Taiko members, personal interview.

61. P. J. Hirabayashi shares "Ei Ja Nai Ka?" internationally as well. In a lecture at the 2015 North American Taiko Conference, she recounted running intensive workshops for Taiko Peace in Bethlehem, where she taught and performed the piece. According to the Web site Taiko Journey, "Aged 12–16, many had never danced or played an instrument in a culture of low self-esteem and oppression, yet all fifty girls found within themselves the strength to learn something from the story of Japanese American pioneers and relate to the universal human bond to our land." http://taikojourney.com/project-partners/taiko-peace-drumming-in-bethlehem/, accessed August 4, 2016.

62. "JACL Continues to Oppose Newly Issued Immigration Ban," September 25, 2017. Press Release, Japanese American Citizens League, https://jacl.org/jacl-continues-opposition-to-newly-issued-immigration-ban/, accessed November 25, 2017.

63. Josephine Lee, *Performing Asian America: Race and Ethnicity on the Contemporary Stage* (Philadelphia: Temple University Press, 1997), 137.

64. Members who performed in this concert, part of the 2009 Rhythm Journey Tour, were Yurika Chiba, P. J. Hirabayashi, Alex Hudson, Franco Imperial, Dylan Solomon, Meg Suzuki, Wisa Uemura, and Adam Weiner.

65. Long Center for the Performing Arts, Austin, Texas, season brochure, author's personal archive, 2009.

66. Susan L. Foster, "Worlding Dance: An Introduction," in *Worlding Dance*, ed. Susan L. Foster (New York: Palgrave Macmillan, 2009), 2.

67. Emily Roxworthy, *The Spectacle of Japanese American Trauma: Racial Performativity and World War II* (Honolulu: University of Hawai'i Press, 2008), 21.

68. Long Center for the Performing Arts season brochure.

69. San Jose Taiko members, personal interview. The following quotations from group members are also from this interview.

CHAPTER 3

1. The phrase "investing in whiteness" comes from George Lipsitz, who argues that the maintenance of whiteness requires both economic and cultural investment. He notes that "social and cultural forces encourage white people to expend time and energy on the creation and re-creation of whiteness." These investments include the accumulation and inheritance of wealth gained through racist policies as well as the preservation of power through

identity. George Lipsitz, *The Possessive Investment in Whiteness: How White People Profit from Identity Politics*, rev. and exp. ed. (Philadelphia: Temple University Press, 2006), vii–viii.

2. Kim Park Nelson, *Invisible Asians: Korean American Adoptees, Asian American Experiences, and Racial Exceptionalism* (New Brunswick: Rutgers University Press, 2016), 13; E. Lee, *Making of Asian America*, 287 (see Chapter 1, n48); "Later Minnesotans," *Minnesota North Star*, November 2, 2009, http://www.state.mn.us/portal/mn/jsp/content.do?id=-8542&subchannel=null&sc2=null&sc3=null&contentid=536879472&contenttype=EDITORIAL&programid=9469&agency=NorthStar.

3. Shimakawa, *National Abjection*, 3–4 (see Chapter 1, n51).

4. This chapter resonates with what Martin F. Manalansan et al. aver in a special issue of *GLQ* on queering the Midwest: that it is important not to "erase the significance of an urban Midwest" and not to draw uncritical demarcations between what is rural and what is urban. Martin F. Manalansan IV et al., "Queering the Middle: Race, Region, and a Queer Midwest," *GLQ: A Journal of Lesbian and Gay Studies*, 20, nos. 1–2 (2014): 3–4.

5. Sun Yung Shin, "Introduction," in *A Good Time for the Truth: Race in Minnesota*, ed. Sun Yung Shin (St. Paul: Minnesota Historical Society Press, 2016), 3.

6. Robin Bernstein, *Racial Innocence: Performing American Childhood from Slavery to Civil Rights* (New York: New York University Press, 2011), 6.

7. Mu Daiko artistic director Jennifer Weir has begun a new nonprofit arts organization, TaikoArts Midwest, which houses two taiko groups: Iris Shiraishi's ensemble-MA and the former Mu Daiko, now named Enso Daiko, under the direction of Weir. Jennifer Weir, pers. comm., July 12, 2016. Mu Performing Arts also announced that it will return to using its original name, Theater Mu.

8. Discover Nikkei, http://www.discovernikkei.org/en/taiko/groups/180/, accessed June 2, 2016.

9. Kogen shares a taiko genealogy with other Buddhist taiko groups across the Midwest and Western states such as Denver Taiko and the Midwest Buddhist Temple in Chicago.

10. Former Mu Daiko member Sara Dejoras formed Misora Daiko in 2002, former members of both Mu Daiko and Kogen Taiko formed Harisen Daiko in 2014, and Iris Shiraishi of Mu Daiko formed ensemble-Ma (or e-MA) in 2015.

11. Rick Shiomi, personal interview, June 18, 2009.

12. Ibid. Shiomi was a founding member of Katari Taiko, Canada's first taiko group. He trained with Seiichi Tanaka at the San Francisco Taiko Dojo during the 1980s while he was developing his play *Yellow Fever* with the Asian American Theatre Company in San Francisco. Shiomi also performed with Wasabi Daiko in Toronto.

13. Jennifer Weir, personal interview, June 28, 2009.

14. Rick Shiomi, personal interview.

15. Ibid.

16. Ibid. Shiomi served as the artistic director of Theater Mu/Mu Performing Arts from 1993 to 2013. He officially oversaw both the taiko and the theatre aspects of the company until 2009, when Iris Shiraishi took over as the taiko programs director, making official a position that she had held in practice for the preceding several years. Shiomi remained artistic director of the company and oversaw the theater component until his retirement in 2013. In 2014, Shiraishi stepped down from her leadership position and from Mu Daiko to pursue other interests; Jennifer Weir served as the artistic director for Mu Daiko from 2015 until September 2017, when Mu Daiko split from Theater Mu.

17. Hsiu-Chen Lin Classon, "A Different Kind of Asian American: Negotiating and Redefining Asian/American in Theater Mu" (PhD diss., Northwestern University, 2000), 229–230. E. K. Lee, *History*, 214 (see Chapter 1, n24). For example, *River of Dreams* and *Legend of the White Snake Lady* incorporated Southeast Asian and Chinese dance,

respectively; Korean mask dance is a key aesthetic element in three plays about Korean adoption (*Mask Dance, Walleye Kid,* and *The Walleye Kid: The Musical*); and renowned Chinese pipa player Gao Hong lent her personal narrative and her pipa talents to *Song of the Pipa.*

18. E. K. Lee, *History,* 215.

19. "Taiko in the USA and Canada USA" (see the preface, n7). People who identify in racial groups other than white or Asian American make up less than 3 percent of survey respondents, including players in the United States and Canada.

20. Iris Shiraishi, Susie Kuniyoshi, Heewon Lee, and Susan Tanabe are a few members who came with musical backgrounds, and Jeff Ellsworth, Rachel Gorton, Drew Gorton, and Al Zdrazil had connections or deep interests in Japan. This is a selective, not an exhaustive, list of Mu Daiko members.

21. Rachel Gorton, personal interview, June 27, 2009.

22. Al Zdrazil, personal interview, June 25, 2009.

23. Susie Kuniyoshi, personal interview, June 19, 2009. All further quotations from Susie Kuniyoshi are from this interview.

24. Su-Yoon Ko, email interview, June 15, 2016; and email communication, July 28, 2017.

25. Mu Performing Arts Outreach Programs, 2009–2010 brochure, personal archive, 2009.

26. Mu Performing Arts Outreach Statistics, internal document, 2009.

27. Shiomi interview, June 18, 2009.

28. Shiomi interview, June 18, 2009. Kogen Taiko, another local ensemble, has also performed in the Twin Cities for many years. Because it only performs when all fifteen members can participate, it does not compete directly with many of the three-person lecture-demonstrations given regularly by Mu Daiko.

29. Vijay Prashad, *Everybody Was Kung Fu Fighting: Afro-Asian Connections and the Myth of Cultural Purity* (Boston: Beacon, 2001), 63. There is no shortage of critiques of multiculturalism in the United States. See also Angela Davis, "Gender, Class, and Multiculturalism," in *Mapping Multiculturalism,* ed. Avery Gordon and Christopher Newfield (Minneapolis: University of Minnesota Press, 1996), 47. Davis writes, "A Multiculturalism that does not acknowledge the political character of culture will not, I am sure, lead toward the dismantling of racist, sexist, homophobic, economically exploitative institutions."

30. Kuniyoshi interview.

31. Diana Taylor, *The Archive and the Repertoire: Performing Cultural Memory in the Americas* (Durham: Duke University Press, 2003), 21.

32. Ibid., 28.

33. Ibid., 54.

34. Outreach brochures from 2008–2009 and earlier play into this exoticizing sentiment in their program description: "From the traditions of ancient China to the powerful stories of Korean adoptees in Minnesota today, Mu Performing Arts outreach performances combine the power and beauty of Asian music and dance with the immediacy of contemporary drama and culture."

35. Heewon Lee, personal interview, June 18, 2009.

36. Taylor, 55.

37. Jeff Ellsworth, personal interview, June 18, 2009.

38. According to its Web site, the group was founded in 2007. For more information about Honoring Women Worldwide, see http://honoringwomenworldwide.net/, accessed December 5, 2017.

39. The grant would provide $75,000 over a period of three years.

40. Shiomi interview, August 8, 2009.

41. Ibid.

42. E. K. Lee, *History*, 26–41.

43. Shiomi interview, August 8, 2009.

44. "Grandmaster Seiichi Tanaka," San Francisco Taiko Dojo Web site, http://www.sftaiko.com/tanaka-1/, April 13, 2017.

45. Shiomi interview, August 8, 2009.

46. Gregg Amundson, personal interview, June 27, 2009.

47. H. Lee interview.

48. The obfuscation of the modern histories of taiko in favor of histories that privilege its ancient past resonates with the ways in which modern dance histories of Bharata Natyam disappear under the weight of its classical status. See Janet O'Shea, *At Home in the World: Bharata Natyam on the Global Stage* (Middletown, CT: Wesleyan University Press, 2007). Similarly, Priya Srinivasan argues that focusing on classical aspects of Indian dance obscures the ways in which modern dance history is rife with Orientalism. See Srinivasan, *Sweating Saris* (see Chapter 1, n29).

49. See also Yoon, " 'She's Really Japanese Now!' " (see the preface, n6), which makes a similar argument about New York's Soh Daiko.

50. At the time of our interview, Shiomi told me that the group was in talks about how to shift the basic outreach framework to address taiko's Asian American roots and issues of race more directly. When race and ethnicity have come up, Shiomi said, they were met with some degree of ambivalence: "Internally in Mu: 'Oh. Oh. Oh. Is that—other things other than just hitting the drum matter?' You know what I mean? And so that whole thing is like starting to shake up the company—Mu Daiko, in a sense." Shiomi interview, August 8, 2009.

51. Taylor, *Archive and the Repertoire*, 58.

52. Weir interview.

53. Iris Shiraishi, personal interview, June 19, 2009.

54. Park Nelson, *Invisible Asians*, 111.

55. Arlie Russell Hochschild, *The Managed Heart: Commercialization of Human Feeling* (Berkeley: University of California Press, 1983), 7.

56. Louwanda Evans and Wendy Leo Moore, "Impossible Burdens: White Institutions, Emotional Labor, and Micro-Resistance," *Social Problems* 62 (2015): 440.

57. Sarah Ahmed, *Living a Feminist Life* (Durham: Duke University Press, 2017), 37.

58. David Roediger, *Towards the Abolition of Whiteness: Essays on Race, Politics, and Working Class History* (London: Verso, 1994), 117–119. Thank you to the anonymous reviewer at Oxford University Press for pointing me toward Roediger's writing about the history of the term *gook* and McCain's usage of it, and further, for urging me to think of the word and the machine-gun gesture as parts of a repertoire of racist gestures that can be deployed in a variety of settings.

59. Ibid.

60. C. W. Nevius et al., "McCain Criticized for Slur: Says he'll keep using the term for ex-captors in Vietnam," *SFGate*, February 18, 2000. http://www.sfgate.com/politics/article/McCain-Criticized-for-Slur-He-says-he-ll-keep-3304741.php, accessed December 6, 2017. In the article, McCain is quoted as saying, "I hate the gooks . . . I will hate them as long as I live." Thank you to the anonymous reviewer from Oxford University Press for pointing me to this incident.

61. Bernstein, *Racial Innocence*, 209–212.

62. David Mura, "A Surrealist History of One Asian American in Minnesota," in *A Good Time for the Truth: Race in Minnesota*, ed. Sun Yung Shin (St. Paul: Minnesota Historical Society Press, 2016), 53–54.

63. Bernstein, *Racial Innocence*, 41.

64. I write on the heels of the acquittal of the officer who shot Philando Castile and the more recent shooting death at police hands of a white woman, Justine Damond. As David Mura writes, Minnesotans' deflection of racism also requires forgetting about "Fong Lee, an unarmed Hmong man shot by police in Minneapolis in 2006. Or Chris Lollie, the black man tasered in the St. Paul skyway in 2014. Or the racial segregation that is still a substantial factor in Minnesota life." See Mura, "Surrealist History," 54.

65. Park Nelson, *Invisible Asians*, 13.

66. Ibid., 96.

67. Ibid., 101.

68. Ibid., 116.

69. Ibid., 140.

70. Stories about Korean adoptees figure prominently in Theater Mu's mainstage and outreach productions. For example, the first play I stage managed for the company in 1998 was *The Walleye Kid*, a play that wove a contemporary story about Korean adoption with a Japanese folk tale. Mu later produced a musical adaptation of the show, and the experiences of two adopted Korean sisters in Minnesota formed the basis for one of Theater Mu's first shows, *Mask Dance*. Katie Hae Leo, an actor and playwright long involved with Mu, wrote *Four Destinies*, which Mu produced as part of its mainstage season in 2011–2012. Further, Sundraya Kase and Sun Mee Chomet, both Korean adoptees, wrote and performed one-woman shows about their experiences, and each was, for several years, part of Theater Mu's outreach offerings. The presence of Korean adoptee players within Mu Daiko, then, reflects both the participation of adoptees in Mu Performing Arts as well as their significant presence within the Asian American population of Minnesota.

71. For an introduction to writings by transnational adoptees, see *Outsiders Within: Writing on Transracial Adoption*, ed. Jane Jeong Trenka, Julia Chinyere Oparah, and Sun Yung Shin. (Cambridge, MA: South End Press, 2006).

72. Josephine Lee, "Introduction," *Asian American Plays for a New Generation*, ed. Josephine Lee, Don Eitel, and R. A. Shiomi (Philadelphia: Temple University Press, 2011), 5.

73. Weir interview.

74. Weir interview.

75. The issue of transnational adoptees' citizenship status made mainstream news after Korean adoptee Adam Crasper was forced to return to South Korea at the age of thirty-seven after living in the United States since he was four years old, when his American parents adopted him. See Alyssa Jeong Perry, "After 37 years in US, Korean adoptee speaks out about imminent deportation," *Guardian*, October 28, 2016; Choe Sang-Hun, "Deportation a 'Death Sentence' to Adoptees after a Lifetime in the US," *New York Times*, July 2, 2017.

76. Jae Ran Kim, "Scattered Seeds: The Christian Influence on Korean Adoption," in *Outsiders Within: Writing on Transracial Adoption*, ed. Jane Jeong Trenka, Julia Chinyere Oparah, and Sun Yung Shin (Cambridge, MA: South End Press, 2006), 153–154. For more perspectives on imperialism and Korean adoption, see Soo Jin Pate, *From Orphan to Adoptee: U.S. Empire and Genealogies of Korean Adoption* (Minneapolis: University of Minnesota Press, 2014).

77. J.R. Kim, "Scattered Seeds," 158.

78. Park Nelson, *Invisible Asians*, 100–103.

79. Su-Yoon Ko, "Reaching," video recording, personal archive.

80. Su-Yoon Ko, "Reaching," manuscript.

81. My use of the term "disidentification" is indebted to José Esteban Muñoz, *Disidentifications: Queers of Color and the Performance of Politics* (Minneapolis: University of Minnesota Press, 1999).

82. Ko, "Reaching," manuscript.

83. Su-Yoon Ko, conversation with the author, June 13, 2017.

CHAPTER 4

1. "Space Heaters," *Life with Bonnie,* with Bonnie Hunt, ABC, (season 2, episode 14), January 30, 2004, VHS recording, personal archive.

2. For a compelling reading of taiko's deployment in *Rising Sun,* see Wong, *Speak It Louder,* 209–214 (see Chapter 1, n4).

3. In his foundational work on whiteness in mainstream film, Richard Dyer demonstrates how whiteness, often configured as normal or natural, becomes visible in certain films that feature nonwhite characters prominently. See his "White," in *The Matter of Images: Essays on Representation,* ed. Richard Dyer (London: Routledge, 1993), 144. See also Peggy Phelan, *Unmarked: The Politics of Performance* (London: Routledge, 1993).

4. For more information about Art Lee and Wadaiko Tokara, see http://www.tokara.net/ArtLee/Artprofile.html.

5. C. Kim, "Racial Triangulation," 106–107 (see Chapter 1, n28).

6. There are other ways to look at data about white women: of women taiko players in the United States, 29 percent are white, whereas in Canada, 33 percent of women taiko players are white. Thank you to Kate Walker for pulling these data points from the TCA Taiko Census 2016. Kate Walker, email to the author, September 6, 2017.

7. Robin DiAngelo, "White Fragility," *International Journal of Critical Pedagogy* 3 (2011): 54–70.

8. Scholarship that addresses casting in Asian American theater studies most often focuses on the musical *Miss Saigon,* in which white British actor Jonathan Pryce played a Eurasian character in yellowface, despite protests by Asian American actors. Yellowface casting controversies arise relatively frequently in American theater, including a Cincinnati production of *Avenue Q* that cast a white actress in the role of Christmas Eve, a first-generation Japanese character. The protest of *Miss Saigon* was not only focused on casting; the play—based on the Orientalist text *Madama Butterfly*—draws deeply on stereotypes of Asians, especially women. For details about the casting and content issues surrounding *Miss Saigon,* see E. K. Lee, *History* (see Chapter 1, n24); J. Lee, *Performing* (see Chapter 2, n63); and Y. Wong, *Choreographing* (see Chapter 1, n29).

9. Scholars in black and Latino/a performance studies have made similar arguments about forms such as gospel music and Latin dance. Drawing on the work of Eric Lott and Michael Rogin, E. Patrick Johnson maintains that blackness does not inhere only in black bodies but that "White Americans also construct blackness." See E. Patrick Johnson, *Appropriating Blackness: Performance and the Politics of Authenticity* (Durham: Duke University Press, 2003), 4. In a similar vein, dance ethnographer Cindy Garcia writes in her study of Los Angeles salsa clubs that both Latinas/os and others construct Latinidad, which, she says, "does not necessarily stick to Latina/o bodies." See Cindy Garcia, *Salsa Crossings: Dancing Latinidad in Los Angeles* (Durham: Duke University Press, 2013), 9. Often, as Johnson notes, constructions of blackness are based on essentialized binary conceptions of whiteness as superior and blackness as inferior, as exemplified by the exaggerated types in blackface minstrelsy. White appropriation of blackness is "an even more complicated dynamic," Johnson writes, one that is never free of "the historical weight of white skin privilege" (4).

10. North American Taiko Conference program, 2003, personal archive.

11. Ibid.

12. Nicole Stansbury, personal interview, June 12, 2015. All subsequent quotations from Stansbury are from this interview.

13. DiAngelo, "White Fragility," 57.

14. Ibid., 58–63.

15. Rachel Gorton, email communication, August 6, 2017.

16. Dyer, "White," 44.

17. John Garvey and Noel Ignatiev, "Toward a New Abolitionism: A *Race Traitor* Manifesto," in *Whiteness: A Critical Reader*, ed. Mike Hill (New York: New York University Press, 1997), 346–347.

18. Rosemary Candelario, *Flowers Cracking Concrete: Eiko and Koma's Asian/American Choreographies* (Middleton, CT: Wesleyan University Press, 2016), 101.

19. I am using the term "social mobility" in a broader way than might be typical in sociology. Rather than referring to white women's ability to rise in education and employment hierarchies, I use the term to indicate that white women can traverse social and cultural spheres in ways not as available to women of color.

20. See Mari Yoshihara, *Embracing the East: White Women and American Orientalism* (New York: Oxford University Press, 2003); Josephine Lee, *The Japan of Pure Invention: Gilbert and Sullivan's* The Mikado (Minneapolis: University of Minnesota Press, 2010).

21. Although part of the chapter is autoethnographic, I interviewed five other women for this chapter, including Rachel Gorton, with whom I performed for a number of years in Mu Daiko in Minneapolis, Minnesota, and Nicole Stansbury, a member of Odaiko Sonora in Tucson, Arizona. They are by no means the only white women taiko players I know; many of the women who took the taiko classes that Mu Daiko offered, for example, are also white, as are many other taiko players. I also interviewed three women who identify, at least in part, as black: Sascha Molina of Sacramento Taiko Dan, Shereen Youngblood of Godaiko Drummers in Northville, Michigan, and Amanda [surname withheld] of Soten Taiko in Des Moines, Iowa.

22. Dyer, "White," 145, 157.

23. Kate Davy, "Outing Whiteness: A Feminist/Lesbian Project," in *Whiteness: A Critical Reader*, ed. Mike Hill (New York: New York University Press, 1997), 211.

24. Ibid., 212–213.

25. Wang, *Soundtracks of Asian America*, 7 (see Chapter 1, n54).

26. Wong, *Speak It Louder*, 216–219.

27. Census data from the TCA indicate that educational level is a commonality among most taiko players. Nearly 90 percent of North American taiko players surveyed indicated that they had at least some college-level educational experience. "Taiko in Canada and the USA" (see the preface, n7).

28. "Introduction," http://www.jetprogramme.org/e/introduction/index.html, December 7, 2010. The Japan Exchange and Teaching Programme began in 1987 with a goal of "promoting grass-roots international exchange between Japan and other nations." According to a chart on its Web site, nearly one-half of its 4,334 current participants from the United States, the largest number from one country. "Current Statistics," December 7, 2010, http://www.jetprogramme.org/e/introduction/statistics.html.

29. Gorton interview (see Chapter 3, n21). All subsequent quotations from Rachel Gorton are from this interview unless otherwise noted. Rachel and Drew Gorton, along with local taiko enthusiast Steve Lein, formed Minnesota Taiko, which built and sold drums to Mu Daiko and other taiko groups throughout the country. See http://www.mntaiko.com/.

30. See also Angela K. Ahlgren, "Futari Tomo: A Queer Duet for Taiko," in *Queer Dance: Meanings and Makings*, ed. Clare Croft (New York: Oxford University Press, 2017), 229–242.

31. Ahlgren, "Futari Tomo."

32. Gorton interview

33. Ruth Frankenberg, *White Women, Race Matters* (Minneapolis: University of Minnesota Press, 1993), 203.

34. Gorton interview.

35. Ibid.

36. When the group invited the four Mu Daiko women members to play, it was after they had seen us perform an all-women's piece, "Naihatsu," by Jennifer Weir, at the 2003 North American Taiko Conference. Rachel Gorton, Iris Shiraishi, Jennifer Weir, and I were part of this concert in May 2005.

37. Amanda [surname withheld], email interview, July 1, 2017. All further quotations by Amanda are from this interview.

38. "Taiko in Canada and the USA."

39. As I noted above, one of the most high-profile African American taiko players is Art Lee, who lives and works in Japan. I also interviewed David Wells, a player who identifies as mixed-race a black man who plays with a number of California taiko groups; and many of his reflections echo Molina's.

40. Kenny Endo, personal interview, March 7, 2014.

41. Nisei (second-generation Japanese Americans) are often characterized by their assimilationist politics, but Diane Fujino points to these and other prominent Nisei activists as exceptions whose activism and familiarity with civil rights and black nationalist politics in the late 1950s and early 1960s helped them become leaders in the Asian American movement. See Fujino, "Race, Space, Place" (see Chapter 1, n16), 57–79.

42. Ibid., 62.

43. Russell Baba, Life History Interview; Roy Hirabayashi, Life History Interview; George Abe, Life History Interview.

44. One notable exception is Reverend Mas Kodani, who acknowledged at a North American Taiko Conference and in his Life History Interview that most North American taiko repertoire is based on Afro-Caribbean rhythms, rather than Japanese music. This accords with the idea of North American taiko as sansei music practice, influenced by American musical styles.

45. Sascha Molina, personal interview, June 13, 2015.

46. "Traditional" practices in taiko might include, for example, the Edo Kotobuki Jishi (Lion Dance), Hachijo drumming from the Hachijo Islands, and Yatai Bayashi, among others.

47. Molina's reference to being a black woman in competitive swimming resonates with August 2016 articles explaining the significance of Simone Manuel's gold medal in swimming. Her victory is particularly meaningful because swimming pools were off-limits to African Americans under Jim Crow.

48. Shereen Youngblood, personal interview, June 29, 2017. All subsequent quotations are from this interview.

49. See C. Kim, "Racial Triangulation of Asian Americans" (see Chapter 1, n28).

50. This sentiment that taiko is a space comparatively free of the racism found in society at large was made explicit by Tanis Sotelo, a Mexican American performer in Iowa. While his compelling interview does not fit within the parameters of this chapter, it is worth noting that he frames taiko as an art form that allows him to avoid and challenge negative stereotypes of Mexican Americans. He says, "I play Taiko today, not only because I enjoy learning about Japanese culture and playing a Japanese instrument, but also [to] make people think of me as [an] artist or musician, rather than think about my race and judge me right away." Tanis Sotelo, email Interview, June 6, 2017.

51. Sunaina Maira, "Belly Dancing: Arab-Face, Orientalist Feminism, and U.S. Empire," *American Quarterly* 60, no. 2 (June 2008): 317–345.

52. Y. Wong, *Choreographing*, 13. Priya Srinivasan makes a related argument about Ruth St. Denis in *Sweating Saris* (see Chapter 1, n29).

53. Bertolt Brecht, "Alienation Effects in Chinese Acting (1935)," in *Theatre/Theory/ Theatre: The Major Critical Texts from Aristotle and Zeami to Soyinka and Havel*, ed. Daniel Gerould (New York: Applause Theatre & Cinema Books, 2000), 460.

54. Anthea Kraut, *Choreographing the Folk: The Dance Stagings of Zora Neale Hurston* (Minneapolis: University of Minnesota Press, 2008), x.

55. Shiraishi interview (see Chapter 3, n53).

56. "About the Center's Namesakes," Lealtad-Suzuki Center, Macalester College, December 16, 2010 http://www.macalester.edu/lealtad-suzuki/about.html.

57. Shiraishi interview.

58. Rachel Gorton, email to the author August 6, 2017.

59. Iris Shiraishi, email to the author.

60. Ibid.

61. I am especially interested in how white women navigate their practice and performance of taiko, given the role white American women have played in adopting Orientalist modes of performance across historical moments, in particular, their art making, self-fashioning, and material consumption from the end of the nineteenth century through the middle of the twentieth. These practices coincided with the enactment of anti-Asian laws and the spread of anti-Asian sentiments throughout the United States. Mari Yoshihara has written about white American women during this time frame who performed Asian theatrical roles such as Cio-Cio-San in *Madama Butterfly* and Maud Allen in *The Darling of the Gods*. While these performers helped shape Orientalist ideas of the age by their perpetuation of Asian female stereotypes, the roles they played also allowed them freedoms that their lives as white, middle-class women denied them. Other women employed Asian literary and visual modes in their artwork in order to claim new expressions of femininity. Although their marginalized status as women allowed them to see "themselves in alliance with the racially oppressed, geopolitically dominated, socioeconomically exploited peoples of the colonies," they also participated in and helped shape the pervasive Orientalism of the era. See Mari Yoshihara *Embracing the East*, 78–79, 6, and 193. Josephine Lee writes that English and American women in the late nineteenth century employed *Mikado*-inspired Japanese goods as a form of safe exoticism that allowed them freedom of expression at a time when their worlds were otherwise strictly limited. See J. Lee, *Japan of Pure Invention*. In her study of modern dance pioneer Ruth St. Denis's Indian-inspired dances, Priya Srinivasan argues that St. Denis's adoption of Asian costumes and choreography was far from innocuous and that it reproduced the racial hierarchies and racist labor practices of her day. See Srinivasan, *Sweating Saris*, 67–102.

62. I align my approach with that of Priya Srinivasan's "unruly spectator," a position she occupies in her book *Sweating Saris* as a scholar who "offers a feminist perspective on spectatorship and takes an active role in uncovering the ways that power can be negotiated" by looking at "mistakes," things that are not supposed to be noticed. Srinivasan, *Sweating Saris*, 16–17.

63. Gorton email.

CHAPTER 5

1. Pride in Art was re-named Queer Arts in 2010. See http://queerartsfestival.com/about-the-queer-arts-festival/pride-in-art-society/.

2. I place the word "traditional" in quotation marks to call attention to the contested nature of this term. What constitutes traditional taiko music is a matter of debate among taiko players. Here, I use "traditional" to signal that a particular song is not an original

composition by the performing group in question. and to indicate that the performances of these pieces in some way stand in relation to an earlier or authoritative version.

3. Queer studies scholars Lauren Berlant and Michael Warner imagine a queer world as "a space of entrances, exits, [and] unsystematized lines of acquaintance" and a space in which intimacies can develop in out-of-the-ordinary ways. Lauren Berlant and Michael Warner, "Sex in Public," *Queer Studies: An Interdisciplinary Reader*, ed. Robert Corber and Stephen Valocchi (Malden, MA: Blackwell, 2003), 175.

4. About a decade after the first two women's groups (Sawagi Taiko and Jodaiko) formed, two more emerged in Toronto and Denver. The Toronto-based RAW (Raging Asian Women), which formed in 1998, describe themselves as "a diverse collective of East and South-East Asian women carrying on the North American taiko drumming tradition and promoting social justice while making music." See http://www.ragingasianwomen.ca/index2.html, accessed March 8, 2011. The promotional materials of Mirai Daiko of Denver, founded in 2002, do not indicate that the choice of being a women's group is connected to any particular political stance. See http://www.miraidaiko.com/live/, accessed March 9, 2011.

5. Y. Wong, *Choreographing*, 41 (see Chapter 1, n29).

6. D. Wong, "Taiko and the Asian/American Body," 74–75 (see the preface, n.7).

7. See Yoon, "Asian Masculinities" (see the preface, n8).

8. Jane Desmond, "Introduction," in *Dancing Desires: Choreographing Sexualities On and Off the Stage*, ed. Jane Desmond (Madison: University of Wisconsin Press, 2001), 17.

9. Clare Croft, "Introduction," in *Queer Dance: Meanings and Makings*, ed. Clare Croft (Ann Arbor: University of Michigan Press, 2017), 4–5.

10. I draw again on Diana Taylor's "scenarios of discovery," oft-repeated scenes of colonial encounter that can nonetheless be changed and repeated through performance. See Taylor, *Archive and the Repertoire*, 28–33 (see Chapter 3, n31).

11. I am influenced in this regard by Alexander Doty, *Making Things Perfectly Queer: Interpreting Mass Culture* (Minneapolis: University of Minnesota Press, 1993).

12. Desmond, "Introduction," 6.

13. Thomas DeFrantz, "Blacking Queer Dance," *Dance Research Journal* 34, no. 2 (2002): 103.

14. Stacy Wolf, *A Problem Like Maria: Gender and Sexuality in the American Musical* (Ann Arbor: University of Michigan Press, 2002), 23.

15. D. Wong, "Taiko and the Asian/American Body," 67–78; Yoon, "'She's Really Become Japanese Now!'" 417–438 (see preface, n6).

16. D. Wong, *Speak it Louder*, 16 (see Chapter 1, n4).

17. Ibid., 219.

18. To avoid repeating the lengthy phrase "Asian, Asian American, and Asian Canadian" each time I describe the group, I use the term "Asian" as shorthand for the range of Asian ethnicities and nationalities of group members. When describing individual players, I strive for specificity. Similarly, I use the term "queer" to refer to the range of ways group members described their sexual identity. Jodaiko members identified their individual sexualities in a range of ways, including lesbian, queer, and gender queer. For one, "queer" signaled a desire to blur the gender binary, while for another, "queer" as a word for nonnormative seemed to be a way to avoid being directly "out" in print. This range points to the heterogeneity within the term "queer" among a given group of people and to the still-high stakes of queer visibility. Finally, one member identified at the time of my research as transgender but was not using male pronouns. Thus, I refer to all members as women and use the pronouns "she/hers."

19. Pachter, *Wadaiko*, (see Chapter 1, n35).

20. Tusler, *Sounds and Sights*, 138 (see Chapter 1, n8).

21. Mercer, Life History Interview.

22. Tusler, *Sounds and Sights*, 138.

23. For a nuanced discussion of San Francisco Taiko Dojo and masculinity, see Yoon, "Asian Masculinities."

24. Tiffany Tamaribuchi, personal interview, October 12, 2009. All further quotations are from this interview unless otherwise specified.

25. As Yoon points out in "Asian Masculinities" (111–112, 126 n16), Tamaribuchi is in some instances the exception to the rule of the SFTD's having excluded women, since she has experienced such success and been included among the top male players in certain performance and teaching situations. On the other hand, she also said in a panel on women and empowerment at NATC 2015 that one male mentor told her he does not think of her as a woman, a statement likely meant as a compliment, reinforcing the high value placed on masculinity.

26. Naomi Guilbert, email to the author, September 22, 2009.

27. The festival, which started in 1976 and ended in 2015, had long been criticized for its exclusion of transgender people. See http://michfest.com/ for information about the festival.

28. Eileen Kage, personal interview, July 31, 2009. All quotations from Eileen Kage are taken from this interview, unless otherwise specified.

29. "History of Sawagi Taiko," Sawagi Taiko Web site. http://www.sawagitaiko.com/files/about_us.htm, accessed August 2, 2016.

30. Leslie Komori, personal interview, August 2, 2009. All quotations from Leslie Komori are taken from this interview, unless otherwise specified.

31. See http://www.taikoelectric.com/about.html.

32. Kristy Oshiro, email to the author, February 2, 2010.

33. There were exceptions to Tamaribuchi's queer-only preference at Pride in Art. In 2006, two straight-identified female members of Mu Daiko appeared as guest artists, and in 2009, Tamaribuchi included two guest artists from Japan who do not identify as queer in the concert lineup. In addition, non-Asian performers have appeared occasionally as guests: in 2006 and 2009, I performed with the group, and white performers Rome Hamner and Nicole Stansbury have also appeared with Jodaiko.

34. North American Taiko Conference program, 2001, personal archive. See also 2003, 2005, 2007, and 2009 programs.

35. North American Taiko Conference program, 2005, personal archive. Whether this division actually happened is questionable, since the leaders report that overall attendance at Curly Noodle sessions had been low until 2009.

36. Yoon, "Asian Masculinities," 123.

37. Kristy Oshiro, email to the author, January 27, 2015.

38. Asian Americans/Pacific Islanders in Philanthropy, "Missed Opportunities: How Organized Philanthropy Can Help Meet the Needs of LGBTQ Asian American, South Asian, Southeast Asian, and Pacific Islander Communities," http://aapip.org/news/2012/01/new-aapip-report-finds-deep-disparities-in-funding-to-lgbtq-aapi-despite-rapidly-growing-population, accessed February 24, 2012.

39. Lowe, *Immigrant Acts*, 66 (see Chapter 1, n58).

40. Sue-Ellen Case, "Toward a Butch-Femme Aesthetic," *The Lesbian and Gay Studies Reader*, ed. Henry Abelove, Michele Barale, and David Halperin (New York: Routledge, 1993), 302.

41. David L. Eng and Alice Y. Hom, "Introduction: Q & A: Notes on a Queer Asian America," *Q & A: Queer in Asian America*, ed. David L. Eng and Alice Y. Hom (Philadelphia: Temple University Press, 1998), 12.

42. See David L. Eng, *Racial Castration: Managing Masculinity in Asian America* (Durham: Duke University Press, 2001).

43. Eng and Hom, "Introduction" 1.

44. Ibid.

45. Wolf, *A Problem Like Maria*, 41–42.

46. Judith (Jack) Halberstam, *Female Masculinity* (Durham: Duke University Press, 1998), 241.

47. Owing to construction, the 2009 Powell Street Festival was relocated to Woodland Park, a few miles from the festival's usual site.

48. Xiaoping Li, "Emergence: Tamio Wakayama" (interview), *Voices Rising: Asian Canadian Cultural Activism* (Vancouver: University of British Columbia Press, 2007), 104.

49. Izumi, "Reconsidering Ethnic Culture," 40–41 (see the preface, n6).

50. Tiffany Tamaribuchi, email to the author, January 28, 2010.

51. "Sensei" is a Japanese word for "teacher." In the context of North American taiko, Tamaribuchi's adoption of the term refers not only to her status as a teacher but also to her status within the groups she leads. That is, whereas some groups operate as a collective without a single leader, Tamaribuchi (like her teacher Seiichi Tanaka) operates her groups based on a hierarchy in which she is the sensei.

52. Toyomi Yoshida, email to the author, January 21, 2010.

53. The reference to being able to breathe freely resonates with the "I Can't Breathe" protests that followed the death of Eric Garner at the hands of New York City police.

54. Eileen Kage, email to the author, September 22, 2009.

55. Tamaribuchi, email to the author.

56. Sharon Holland, *The Erotic Life of Racism* (Durham: Duke University Press, 2012), 46.

57. Richard Dyer, "White," *Screen* 29.4 (1988): 44–64.

58. Dorinne Kondo, "(Un)Disciplined Subjects: (De)Colonizing the Academy?" in *Orientations: Mapping Studies in the Asian Diaspora*, ed. Kandice Chuh and Karen Shimakawa (Durham: Duke University Press, 2001), 32.

59. Celine Parreñas Shimizu, *The Hypersexuality of Race: Performing Asian/American Women on Screen and Scene* (Durham: Duke University Press, 2007), 5.

60. Albright, *Choreographing Difference,* xxii (see the preface, n10).

61. For detailed discussions of the o-daiko and masculinity, see Shawn Bender, "Drumming from Screen to Stage: Ondekoza's Odaiko and the Reimaging of Japanese Taiko," *Journal of Asian Studies* 69, no. 3 (2010): 843–867, and Yoon, "Asian Masculinities."

62. In this tradition, the soloist's performance of "O-daiko" is most often followed immediately by an ensemble piece called "Yatai Bayashi," a song in which the soloist joins several other drummers who perform in a physically demanding sit-up position. Many taiko groups perform versions of these pieces, which are considered part of the public domain, but it is considered good etiquette to secure permission and training from sanctioned teachers before performing them.

63. I have seen Tamaribuchi perform on the o-daiko countless times, both live and on recordings. Although I refer here, in a short ethnographic description, to being in the audience at the 2009 Vancouver Pride in Art festival, my analysis is shaped by the other performances. Most often, I have seen her perform with the hairstyle and costuming I have described here, but I have also seen her perform with long hair and wearing a happi coat. While my analysis is inevitably shaped by all of these events, major sources for this detailed description of Tamaribuchi's physical appearance are a video recording from a performance at the Southern Theater in Minneapolis, Minnesota, in 2006, and my ethnographic research from 2009.

64. Wong, *Speak It Louder*, 218.

65. Bender, "Drumming from Screen to Stage," 860. In "Asian Masculinities," Yoon expresses doubt that Cardin invented the idea of wearing fundoshi on stage, but nonetheless, as he

writes, "the Oriental male body is on display . . . and it is a body that is both exotic (regardless of who initiated this practice) and physically impressive" (108).

66. Bender, "Drumming from Screen to Stage," 861–862.
67. See also Yoon, "Asian Masculinities," 108.
68. Ibid.
69. Ramón H. Rivera-Servera, "Choreographies of Resistance: Latina/o Queer Dance and the Utopian Performative," *Modern Drama* 47, no. 2 (Summer 2004) : 279.
70. Ibid.,271.
71. Quoted in ibid., 278.
72. Jill Dolan, *Utopia in Performance: Finding Hope at the Theater* (Ann Arbor: University of Michigan Press, 2005), 31.
73. For a discussion of taiko's activist and ethnic community roots in Canada, see Izumi, "Reconsidering Ethnic Culture and Community"; on the ties between San Jose Taiko and Asian American activism, see Chapter 2.
74. R.A.W., http://www.ragingasianwomen.ca/index2.html, March 8, 2011.
75. The Genki Spark, www.thegenkispark.org, August 3, 2016.
76. Kristy Oshiro, Queer Taiko classes, http://www.meetup.com/queertaiko/, December 4, 2017.

CONCLUSION

1. Tiffany Tamaribuchi, email to the author, September 4, 2017. All quotations from Tamaribuchi in this chapter are from this communication.
2. In 2014, FBI data showed that 201 people of Asian descent were victims of hate crimes, or 6.2 percent of the 3,227 victims tracked. This accounts only for incidents reported to the FBI. Table 1, "2014 Hate Crime Statistics," Federal Bureau of Investigation Uniform Crime Reporting, https://ucr.fbi.gov/about-us/cjis/ucr/hate-crime/2014/topic-pages/victims_final, accessed July 26, 2016.
3. J. Lee, "Introduction," 5 (see Chapter 3, n72).
4. Taylor, 58 (see Chapter 3, n31).

SELECTED BIBLIOGRAPHY

Ahlgren, Angela K. "Futari Tomo: A Queer Duet for Taiko." In *Queer Dance: Meanings and Makings*, edited by Clare Croft, 229–242. New York: Oxford University Press, 2017.

Ahlgren, Angela K. "A New Taiko Folk Dance: San Jose Taiko and Asian American Movements." In *Contemporary Directions in Asian American Dance*, edited by Yutian Wong, 29–61. Madison: University of Wisconsin Press, 2016.

Ahmed, Sarah. *Living a Feminist Life*. Durham: Duke University Press, 2017.

Asai, Susan. "Horaku: A Buddhist Tradition of Performing Arts and the Development of Taiko Drumming in the United States." *Selected Reports in Ethnomusicology* 6 (1985): 163–172.

Azuma, Eiichiro. *Between Two Empires: Race, History, and Transnationalism in Japanese America*. Oxford: Oxford University Press, 2005.

Bender, Shawn. *Taiko Boom: Japanese Drumming in Place and Motion*. Berkeley: University of California Press, 2012.

Bernstein, Robin. *Racial Innocence: Performing American Childhood from Slavery to Civil Rights*. New York: New York University Press, 2011.

Butler, Judith. "Performative Acts and Gender Constitution: An Essay in Phenomenology and Feminist Theory." *Theatre Journal* 40, no. 4 (December 1988): 519–531.

Candelario, Rosemary. *Flowers Cracking Concrete: Eiko and Koma's Asian/American Choreographies*. Middleton, CT: Wesleyan University Press, 2016.

Canning, Charlotte. "Feminist Performance as Feminist Historiography." *Theatre Survey* 45, no. 2 (November 2004): 227–233.

Croft, Clare. "Introduction." In *Queer Dance: Meanings and Makings*, edited by Clare Croft, 1–33. Ann Arbor: University of Michigan Press, 2017.

Davy, Kate. "Outing Whiteness: A Feminist/Lesbian Project." In *Whiteness: A Critical Reader*, edited by Mike Hill, 204–225. New York: New York University Press, 1997.

DeFrantz, Thomas. "Blacking Queer Dance." *Dance Research Journal* 34, no. 2 (2002): 102–105.

Desmond, Jane, ed. *Dancing Desires: Choreographing Sexualities On and Off the Stage*. Madison: University of Wisconsin Press, 2001.

DiAngelo, Robin. "White Fragility." *International Journal of Critical Pedagogy* 3 (2011): 54–70.

Dolan, Jill. *Utopia in Performance: Finding Hope at the Theater*. Ann Arbor: University of Michigan Press, 2005.

Eng, David L. *Racial Castration: Managing Masculinity in Asian America*. Durham: Duke University Press, 2001.

Eng, David L., and Alice Y. Hom. "Introduction: Q & A: Notes on a Queer Asian America." In *Q & A: Queer in Asian America*, edited by David L. Eng and Alice Y. Hom, 1–21. Philadelphia: Temple University Press, 1998.

Evans, Louwanda, and Wendy Leo Moore. "Impossible Burdens: White Institutions, Emotional Labor, and Micro-Resistance." *Social Problems* 62 (2015): 439–454.

Foster, Susan L., ed. *Worlding Dance*. New York: Palgrave Macmillan, 2009.

Fujino, Diane. "Race, Space, Place and Political Development: Japanese-American Radicalism in the 'Pre-Movement' 1960s." *Social Justice* 35, no. 2 (2008): 57–79.

Garcia, Cindy. *Salsa Crossings: Dancing Latinidad in Los Angeles*. Durham: Duke University Press, 2013.

Halberstam, Judith. *Female Masculinity*. Durham: Duke University Press, 1998.

Hamera, Judith. *Dancing Communities: Performance, Difference, and Connection in the Global City*. New York: Palgrave Macmillan, 2007.

Hochschild, Arlie Russell. *The Managed Heart: Commercialization of Human Feeling*. Berkeley: University of California Press, 1983.

Izumi, Masumi. "Reconsidering Ethnic Culture and Community: A Case Study on Japanese Canadian Taiko Drumming." *Journal of Asian American Studies* 4 (2001): 35–56.

Jones, Joni L. "Performance Ethnography: The Role of Embodiment in Cultural Authenticity." *Theatre Topics* 12, no. 1 (2002): 1–15.

Kim, Claire Jean. "The Racial Triangulation of Asian Americans." *Politics & Society* 27, no. 1 (March 1999): 105–138.

Kim, Jae Ran. "Scattered Seeds: The Christian Influence on Korean Adoption." In *Outsiders Within: Writing on Transracial Adoption*, edited by Jane Jeong Trenka, Julia Chinyere Oparah, and Sun Yung Shin, 151–162. Cambridge, MA: South End Press, 2006.

King, Rebecca Chiyoko. "Multiraciality Reigns Supreme? Mixed-Race Japanese Americans and the Cherry Blossom Queen Pageant." *Amerasia Journal* 23, no. 1 (1997): 116.

Konagaya, Hideo. "Taiko as Performance: Creating Japanese American Traditions." *Japanese Journal of American Studies* 12 (2001): 105–124.

Kondo, Dorinne. "(Un)Disciplined Subjects: (De)Colonizing the Academy?" In *Orientations: Mapping Studies in the Asian Diaspora*, edited by Kandice Chuh and Karen Shimakawa, 25–40. Durham: Duke University Press, 2001.

Kraut, Anthea. *Choreographing the Folk: The Dance Stagings of Zora Neale Hurston*. Minneapolis: University of Minnesota Press, 2008.

Lee, Erika. *The Making of Asian America: A History*. New York: Simon & Schuster, 2015.

Lee, Esther Kim. *A History of Asian American Theatre*. Cambridge: Cambridge University Press, 2006.

Lee, Josephine. "Introduction." In *Asian American Plays for a New Generation*, edited by Josephine Lee, Don Eitel, and R. A. Shiomi, 1–10. Philadelphia: Temple University Press, 2011.

Lee, Josephine. *The Japan of Pure Invention: Gilbert and Sullivan's The Mikado*. Minneapolis: University of Minnesota Press, 2010.

Lee, Josephine. *Performing Asian America: Race and Ethnicity on the Contemporary Stage*. Philadelphia: Temple University Press, 1997.

Li, Xiaoping. "Emergence: Tamio Wakayama" (interview). In *Voices Rising: Asian Canadian Cultural Activism*. Vancouver, 89–106. University of British Columbia Press, 2007.

Lipsitz, George. *The Possessive Investment in Whiteness: How White People Profit from Identity Politics*, rev. expanded ed. Philadelphia: Temple University Press, 2006.

Liu, Michael, Kim Geron, and Tracy A. M. Lai. *The Snake Dance of Asian American Activism: Community, Vision, and Power*. Lanham, MD: Lexington Books, 2008.

Louie, Steve. "When We Wanted It Done, We Did It Ourselves." In *Asian Americans: The Movement and the Moment*, edited by Steve Louie and Glenn K. Omatsu, xv–xxv. Los Angeles: UCLA Asian American Studies Center Press, 2001.

Lowe, Lisa. *Immigrant Acts: On Asian American Cultural Politics*. Durham: Duke University Press, 1996.

Maira, Sunaina. "Belly Dancing: Arab-Face, Orientalist Feminism, and U.S. Empire." *American Quarterly* 60, no. 2 (June 2008): 317–345.

Matsue, Jennifer Milioto. "Drumming to One's Own Beat: Japanese Taiko and the Challenge to Genre." *Ethnomusicology* 60, no. 1 (Winter 2016): 22–52.

Mura, David. "A Surrealist History of One Asian American in Minnesota." In *A Good Time for the Truth: Race in Minnesota*, edited by Sun Yung Shin, 43–58. St. Paul: Minnesota Historical Society Press, 2016.

Okihiro, Gary. "Acting Japanese." In *Japanese Diasporas: Unsung Pasts, Conflicting Presents and Uncertain Futures*, edited by Nobuko Adachi, 191–201. New York: Routledge, 2006.

Omatsu, Glen. "'Four Prisons' and the Movements of Liberation: Asian American Activism from the 1960s to the 1990s." In *Asian American Studies: A Reader*, edited by Jean Yu-wen Shen Wu and Min Song, 164–196. New Brunswick: Rutgers University Press, 2000.

Pachter, Benjamin. "Wadaiko *in Japan and the United States: The Intercultural History of a Musical Genre*." PhD diss., University of Pittsburgh, 2013.

Park Nelson, Kim. *Invisible Asians: Korean American Adoptees, Asian American Experiences, and Racial Exceptionalism*. New Brunswick: Rutgers University Press, 2016.

Rahaim, Matthew. *Musicking Bodies: Gesture and Voice in Hindustani Music*. Middletown, CT: Wesleyan University Press, 2012.

Rivera-Servera, Ramón. *Performing Queer Latinidad: Dance, Sexuality, Politics*. Ann Arbor: University of Michigan Press, 2012.

Roediger, David. *Towards the Abolition of Whiteness: Essays on Race, Politics, and Working Class History*. London: Verso, 1994.

Roxworthy, Emily. *The Spectacle of Japanese American Trauma: Racial Performativity and World War II*. Honolulu: University of Hawai'i Press, 2008.

Schechner, Richard. *Performance Studies: An Introduction*. London: Routledge, 2002.

Shimakawa, Karen. *National Abjection: The Asian American Body Onstage*. Durham: Duke University Press, 2002.

Small, Christopher. *Musicking: The Meanings of Performing and Listening*. Middletown, CT: Wesleyan University Press, 1998.

Srinivasan, Priya. *Sweating Saris: Indian Dance as Transnational Labor*. Philadelphia: Temple University Press, 2012.

Takahashi, Jere. *Nisei/Sansei: Shifting Japanese Identities and Politics*. Philadelphia: Temple University Press, 1997.

Takaki, Ronald. *Strangers from a Different Shore: A History of Asian Americans*, rev. ed. Boston: Little, Brown, 1998.

Taylor, Diana. *The Archive and the Repertoire: Performing Cultural Memory in the Americas*. Durham: Duke University Press, 2003.

Tusler, Mark. "Sounds and Sights of Power: Ensemble Taiko Drumming (Kumi Daiko) Pedagogy in California and the Conceptualization of Power." PhD diss. University of California, Santa Barbara, 2003.

Wang, Grace. *Soundtracks of Asian America: Navigating Race through Musical Performance*. Durham: Duke University Press, 2015.

Wei, William. *The Asian American Movement*. Philadelphia: Temple University Press, 1993.

Wishkoski, Rachel. "'To Become Something New Yet Familiar': Remembering, Moving, and Re-membering in Seattle Buddhist Church's Bon Odori Festival." MA thesis, Ohio State University, 2014.

Wolf, Stacy. *A Problem Like Maria: Gender and Sexuality in the American Musical*. Ann Arbor: University of Michigan Press, 2002.

Wong, Deborah. "Moving: From Performance to Performative Ethnography and Back Again." In *Shadows in the Field: New Perspectives for Fieldwork in Ethnomusicology*, 2nd ed., edited by Gregory Barz and Timothy J. Cooley, 76–89. New York: Oxford University Press, 2008.

Wong, Deborah. *Speak It Louder: Asian Americans Making Music.* New York: Routledge, 2004.

Wong, Deborah. "Taiko and the Asian/American Body: Drums, *Rising Sun,* and the Question of Gender." *World of Music* 42, no. 3 (2000): 67–78.

Wong, Yutian. "Introduction." In *Contemporary Directions in Asian American Dance,* edited by Yutian Wong, 3–26. Madison: University of Wisconsin Press, 2016.

Wong, Yutian. *Choreographing Asian America.* Middletown, CT: Wesleyan University Press, 2010.

Yoon, Paul Jong-Chul. "Asian Masculinities and Parodic Possibilities in Odaiko Solos and Filmic Representations." *Asian Music* 40, no. 1 (2009): 100–130.

Yoon, Paul Jong-Chul. "'She's Really Become Japanese Now!' Taiko Drumming and Asian American Identifications." *American Music* (Winter 2001): 417–438.

Yoshihara, Mari. *Embracing the East: White Women and American Orientalism.* New York: Oxford University Press, 2003.

INDEX